TRANSCENDENTAL MEDITATION

A Scientist's Journey to
Happiness, Health, and Peace

ALSO BY ROBERT KEITH WALLACE

An Introduction to Transcendental Meditation
(with Lincoln Norton)

Maharishi AyurVeda and Vedic Technology
(Physiology of Consciousness: Part 2)

The Neurophysiology of Enlightenment

Dharma Parenting (with Fred Travis)

Dharma Health and Beauty
(with Samantha Wallace)

TRANSCENDENTAL MEDITATION
A Scientist's Journey to
Happiness, Health, and Peace

Adapted and Updated from
The Physiology of Consciousness: Part I

Robert Keith Wallace, PhD

Dharma Publications

ISBN 978-0-9972207-1-1

Library of Congress Control Number: 2016901662

www.DharmaPublications.com

Dharma Publications, Fairfield, IA

Contents

TO
MAHARISHI MAHESH YOGI

Introduction

Discovering Our Inner Physiology

It had taken more than three years of research to prepare for the day I walked down the dimly lit underground corridor that led to the historic Thorndike Memorial Laboratory. The high standards of science practiced in this building were at odds with their surroundings. The Thorndike lab is situated in Boston City Hospital, a network of old, decaying buildings that might be mistaken for a foundling home out of a Dickens novel. Outside was what had become the worst of Boston ghettos. However, I was quickly given to understand that, as a medical researcher, I should take Puritan pride in the dingy setting—it was a badge of honor.

My heart pounded as I walked into the small lecture hall crowded with senior research scientists and medical doctors, the elite of Boston's medical community. I was not worried about the topic of my lecture, which was my PhD thesis research. What was going to be difficult to communicate was the implications of that research. For the first time, a fourth state of consciousness, different from waking, dreaming, and sleeping—a state of pure consciousness—was readily accessible to science. This enormous breakthrough had been made possible by the introduction of an entirely new technology, a technology of consciousness. This technology, the Transcendental Meditation technique of Maharishi Mahesh Yogi, systematically produced in those who practiced it the repeatable experience of pure consciousness. Studying the objective, physiological correlates of Transcendental Meditation, scientists could thus begin to pinpoint the physiology of consciousness.

I wanted this audience to understand that this was a turning point in the history of mankind. Two divergent streams of knowledge were converging. On the one hand, through the objective approach of modern science we were delving into the deepest layers of life and matter. In physiology, we had made enormous breakthroughs in our understanding of the relationship between mind and body. In physics we were on the verge of arriving at a single unified theory of matter and energy—Einstein's great dream. On the other hand, through a new subjective approach to gaining knowledge, we had for the first time a reliable and systematic means to explore the finest levels of our consciousness.

This subjective approach had been brought to light from the timeless Vedic tradition by Maharishi and was proving to be of immense importance to the scientific community. This approach and the new technology of consciousness it offered would entirely change our way of thinking about health and the human body.

The new area of research I was describing that day revealed that underlying our manifest, material physiology is a more fundamental, unmanifest physiology of consciousness. Understanding the physiology of consciousness gives us a new way of understanding and achieving ideal health, not only for the individual, but also for the whole society.

The Biochemistry of Mind

My lecture at Thorndike Memorial Laboratory took place in 1971, at a time when mind-body research was rapidly developing. Since then enormous changes have taken place, both in my own areas of research and in many others. Critical studies, especially in biochemistry, have helped uncover the connections between mind and body.

We can think of the body as having its own natural pharmacy. When we have a thought or feeling, the body responds by producing chemicals. These chemicals, which are produced in numerous types of cells, act as natural drugs that are involved in many different kinds of physiological and behavioral responses. One of the most interesting and widely publicized discoveries is that our mind can instruct our body to produce its own internal painkillers—a group of small protein compounds, or neuropeptides—called endorphins and enkephalins.

For many years researchers have been trying to find the cause of morphine and heroin addiction. In the course of their research, they isolated a particular receptor that seems specifically designed for morphine-type drugs. Receptors are biological molecules embedded on the surface of a cell. Specific hormones or chemicals in the blood and fluid surrounding the cell fit into specific receptors, the way a key fits into a lock. This sets off a chain of events inside the cell that results in a specific physiological action, such as an increase in metabolism.

The morphine molecule fits into certain receptors in the cells of the nervous system which, when activated, greatly reduce pain. Since morphine is a painkiller not normally present in the body, one could reasonably assume that nature designed these receptors for a substance that does exist in the body. That is to say, the body must have its own natural painkiller. Pursuing this logic, researchers were indeed able to identify painkillers produced by the body and to map their pathways throughout the brain and physiology. These painkillers, endorphins and enkephalins, also play a number of other important roles as "biological communicators." One of their most significant roles is to initiate the placebo effect.

A placebo induces the expectation of a pleasing effect, such as relief from pain, and this expectation itself causes the patient to actually experience less pain. It is well known that when subjects in an experiment are told they are being given a new painkilling drug and are instead given a white sugar pill with no active painkilling ingredient—a placebo—a large proportion of these people will not feel any pain, even when subjected to a moderately painful stimulus. For many years no one had any reasonable explanation for how the placebo worked—it was in fact considered a nuisance to scientific research, making it necessary to include more control subjects.

Experiments suggest that the placebo effect is an important scientific breakthrough vividly illustrating the power of the mind over the body. The findings suggest that, in the placebo effect, the mind—convinced it will not feel pain—causes the nervous system to produce endorphins and enkephalins. The result is similar to taking a painkilling drug. One of the most interesting findings about endorphins and enkephalins is that their receptors have been located not only in the nervous system, where we generally think of pain and emotions as being processed, but in many other cells (for example, in the cells of the immune system).

We may consider the neuropeptide molecule and its cousin, the neurotransmitter, to be "precipitated thoughts." If we have an excited thought, then a molecule such as adrenaline arises and stimulates various parts of the body. If we have a calm, soothing thought, then a "calm" molecule arises—that is, one that produces a restful effect on the body. Such molecules form an information network through which any part of the body can "talk" to any other part. From this perspective, our body is a thinking body, in which information or intelligence constantly flows among all its innumerable parts.

This gives rise to the concept of an entirely subjective physiology of consciousness, which underlies our objective physiology of matter. The connection between the two is at the molecular level, where thoughts are translated into chemical messengers. Moment by moment the body is being influenced and changed—is actually being created—by the fluctuations of consciousness projected in our thoughts and feelings. Understood in this way, the mind-body connection has countless ramifications for biomedical research and practice, including the treatment of pain and serious disease.

The Discovery of the Unified Field of All the Laws of Nature

The achievements in mind-body research have paralleled breakthroughs in modern physics. In physics, matter and energy are viewed as expressions of four fundamental fields: gravity, electromagnetism, and the strong and weak nuclear forces. While the complete mathematical description of a unified field is still developing, it is clear that such a field exists as the source of all material diversity. It transcends all existence; it is a field of pure information from which all the different forces and laws of nature sequentially emerged in the first microseconds of the creation of our universe, and from which this process is continually taking place at every moment.

This concept of one unified field of the laws of nature at the basis of creation is found in many cultural traditions of both East and West. In the Vedic tradition of India, all the diversity of material existence has always been described as sequentially emerging from a unified field, a self-sufficient, self-referral, unbounded and infinitely dynamic field of consciousness. As we will see, in the Vedic tradition this unified field is, in fact, defined as a field of pure intelligence, pure information in its most compact and concentrated form—one unified basis of life.

With the advent of modern science some three hundred years ago, these ancient ideas lost their prominence and were eventually displaced by the classical view of physics—the classical paradigm. According to Newtonian classical physics, the world is made of tiny, indestructible atoms. Matter is solid and easily measured. This viewpoint permeated every academic discipline and every area of society, and had an enormous impact on the world-view.

With the development of quantum physics, the classical paradigm has been gradually replaced by the quantum paradigm. In the world of quantum physics, matter is no longer solid; it is only a perturbation, a condensation in an underlying field.

But do these principles ultimately have meaning for human life? One could argue that they make no sense because they have no relation to the "real world" of our everyday lives. Yet according to modern physics, the quantum world is more fundamental than the classical world. We can think of the foundation of a house, hidden from view beneath the ground. Without this foundation, the house cannot stand. The quantum world is the foundation of the classical world. Without the quantum world, the classical world would not exist.

Further, the radical concepts of quantum physics, while defying our sensory experience and rational explanations of the world, give us access to new realms of applied technology. Quantum principles are an essential part of our computer and electronic age. They make possible the miracles of modern technology and reveal the hidden, underlying power and intelligence stored within matter. Matter has thus given way to information. It is easy to understand why it has taken so long for these ideas to be introduced to the general public—they challenged the belief in matter. They broke the boundaries of the classical paradigm and presented reality from an entirely different viewpoint.

A Technology of Consciousness

When I stood before my audience at Thorndike Memorial Laboratory I knew it would be nearly impossible to communicate the importance and impact of this research. As the quantum paradigm led to the introduction of radically new and more powerful technologies at the electronic and nuclear layers of matter, the Transcendental Meditation program would lead to the opening of the realm of consciousness.

In the lecture I presented my first studies on the Transcendental Meditation technique. I had been studying the objective correlates of Transcendental Meditation, attempting to physiologically define the fourth major state of consciousness—transcendental or pure consciousness. While there are many techniques of meditation and self-development, my research had shown conclusively that Transcendental Meditation was the most systematic and reliable for producing consistent physiological correlates of pure consciousness.

In presenting the results of my research to this audience, I realized that to them, the existence of transcendental consciousness could only be appreciated and understood in terms of its objective physiological correlates—heart rate, blood lactate, skin resistance. Yet I knew that, exciting as these findings were, they were only the shadowy reflections of the incomparable richness of the transcendental field of life—the deep mechanics of the laws of nature unfolding within pure consciousness, reverberating unsuspected within these very doctors' own consciousness.

If the real nature of life is a unified field of consciousness, why don't we experience it as the reality of our daily lives? Why do we experience the world as being made of separate material objects: why does our body, for example, appear to be localized in time and space? The reason is that our senses are highly selective. The senses are activated by a narrow spectrum of data from the immense flux of nature, and it is from a selection of that narrow spectrum that our understanding of physical reality is determined.

Our nervous system constructs our reality. The nervous system analyzes the world in terms of patterns of sight, sound, taste, touch, and smell, and then our mind and intellect actively reconstruct within the brain our individual perception of reality. The reason we experience the world from a classical perspective, in which matter appears solid, is that we do not have access to the deeper levels of reality beyond the obvious sensory level of experience.

We have not learned to use the full potential of our nervous system to directly experience and explore the wide range of nature's intelligence; we have been forced to rely on the vision provided for us by objective technology alone. This limited awareness, using only objective means, has led us to know only the grosser aspects of our physiology of matter, which embody a tiny fraction of the laws of nature.

To gain a true picture of the world, we must first use the full abilities of the nervous system to experience consciousness in its simplest state, the state of pure consciousness, the unified field of all the laws of nature. Through the Transcendental Meditation program, the focus of attention is periodically shifted inward. We begin to use our nervous system as a special kind of microscope with which to explore pure consciousness in a systematic and reliable way. This experience cultures our nervous system to function in a more integrated and coherent style.

As a natural and spontaneous result of this experience, our preconditioned interpretation of the world—and the belief system we have built from it—begins to change. With the regular, direct experience of the unified field, our conscious experience and intellect are no longer restricted by the belief that matter is the only reality. We experience a new reality, of pure consciousness at the basis of matter.

We know this, not intellectually but through direct experience. We know it first as the field of pure consciousness at the basis of our own mind. As our practice of these technologies advances, we develop toward higher states of consciousness, and come to know pure consciousness as the field underlying everything we encounter through our senses in the world around us. Our nervous system then constructs for us a reality far richer, more delightful and fulfilling than the one we were accustomed to when the classical viewpoint dominated our sensory experience. Eventually we gain access within our own consciousness to the source of nature's creativity, the dynamic processes that structure the universe. We are no longer separate from nature. As consciousness becomes fully developed, we can look forward to experiencing our inner Self as the consciousness of the universe.

These were the ideas I attempted to express in my lecture so many years ago. If we are able to experience the full range of consciousness, the restrictions on our awareness are removed: we transcend the myth of matter and gain a complete and unified understanding of life.

CHAPTER 1

The Anatomy of Consciousness

In 1974 I flew with a physicist friend to Nepal. We made our way up from Katmandu, the capital, to be nearer the Himalayas, and found a beautiful alpine lake, which Nepalese princes once favored as a summer retreat. For less than a dollar, we rented a small boat and pushed out onto the water. It was a windy day with clearing skies, a perfect day to fly kites. I had bought one at the bazaar. It was painted a fierce red and built for acrobatics. As I stood up in the boat and let the kite loose on the wind, it jumped from my hand. Children ran along the shore, laughing and waving to us. The kite floated high into the thin air. I remember looking up toward the great mountains around us. Though they were mostly covered with clouds, they gave off an aura of grandeur and peace. I felt content, almost drowsy, in this moment of ease. As I watched, the clouds lifted all at once. I was absolutely in awe. What I had taken for mountains were only foothills! Beyond, like ancient gods, rose the true Himalayas, unbelievably mighty and majestic.

So much power and beauty were concentrated in that breathtaking scene that my friend and I could hardly speak. The name of one of the tallest peaks is Annapurna, which means "fullness of life." And what I experienced in that moment was a feeling of utter fulfillment and unboundedness, a simple yet profound conviction that time really is timeless, and that anything is possible.

The Himalayas are the home of the Vedic tradition of India, and people have always journeyed there seeking enlightenment. In the Vedic tradition, enlightenment represents the ultimate development of what we consider the most valuable qualities of human life. It is something real and natural. It develops continuously, progressively, and systematically on the basis of neurophysiological refinement utilizing the full potential of human physiology.

Throughout the world I have found a genuine interest, among serious scientists and laypeople alike, in consciousness and enlightenment. Everywhere, there is the growing recognition that we have neglected the subjective development of life and have become too obsessed with material development. We understand in great detail the anatomy of matter; it is now time to focus on the anatomy of consciousness.

Pure Consciousness

What we consider to be ordinary waking consciousness is a very restricted value of the full range of human consciousness. It corresponds with the more active levels of human life. Systematically quieting the internal functioning of the physiology while enlivening the deeper levels of mental awareness allows us to experience the fourth state of consciousness—a much fuller and more universal state of consciousness—one that is completely awake, yet settled and unified.

This unified state of consciousness is referred to as transcendental consciousness. It is the experience of pure consciousness, the unified field of all the laws of nature, the transcendental field of life. To experience this state, our attention has been brought from the active, surface level of everyday thinking to the silent, unbounded ocean of consciousness at the basis of the mind. In the experience of pure consciousness, there are no thoughts, no sensory experience, and no distinction between subject and object—only pure awareness, the experience of consciousness knowing itself.

When you see any object—a rose, for instance—there are three modes of your experience. There is you, the knower; the rose, the known; and the connection between you and the rose, the processes of perception or knowing. This structure works differently in waking consciousness, however, from the way it does in the state of pure consciousness. When you experience the rose in waking consciousness, your awareness becomes identified with it, and the knower becomes overshadowed. Only the rose, the object of knowing, is lively in your experience. In higher states of consciousness we still experience the rose in all its glory but the experience of the rose no longer overshadows our underlying experience of pure consciousness, pure awareness.

The goal of higher states of consciousness is to enliven this unified state of consciousness, the unified field of all the laws of nature, in our own awareness using specific mental technologies, so that the fundamental laws governing human physiology and all of life everywhere become fully lively in our life. This possibility has tremendous implications for the fields of psychology, physiology, and the health sciences; as we shall see later on, it is the basis for creating ideal health for the individual and ideal health for the whole society—a state of irreversible world peace.

Higher States of Consciousness

The regular experience of pure consciousness refines our physiology of matter so that we are able to realize the full range of human development in higher states of consciousness.

Our understanding and experience of consciousness itself has been limited, because we have had access to only three states of consciousness: waking, dreaming, and sleeping. The Vedic tradition delineates distinct higher states of consciousness and describes precisely how they develop through regular practice of the Transcendental Meditation program. If we don't have the tools to develop and experience higher states of consciousness, then we confine ourselves to an extremely limited experience and understanding of nature; we isolate ourselves from the very heart of our own existence.

Maharishi gave us the understanding and experience of seven states of consciousness—the three we are all familiar with, plus pure consciousness and three distinct higher states. The first step toward higher states of consciousness is to experience the fourth state—pure consciousness. With the regular experience of pure consciousness during Transcendental Meditation, the nervous system adapts to a new style of functioning. The alternation of transcendental consciousness with the regular daily cycle of waking activity, dreaming, and sleep produces a gradual refinement of neurophysiological functions. This results in a fifth state of consciousness—a new, more expanded state known as cosmic consciousness.

In cosmic consciousness the individual realizes his essential identity as transcendental or pure consciousness as an all-time reality. In this fifth state, transcendental consciousness coexists with waking, dreaming, and sleep. For example, in cosmic consciousness, even in the most dynamic waking-state activity, one has an inner quality of consciousness that is restful and absolutely clear; even while sleeping, one experiences the inner alertness of transcendental consciousness. Maharishi refers to this all-time silent inner alertness, which is the experience of transcendental consciousness along with all the changing states of awareness, as "witnessing."

In cosmic consciousness, because the awareness is permanently established in the field of pure consciousness, the impressions made by an object upon the nervous system no longer overshadow the knower. An analogy may help explain this. In ordinary waking consciousness, our experience of anything in the outside world—even a beautiful rose—is like etching a line in rock: it leaves a deep, long-lasting impression that is difficult to erase and overshadows the underlying nature of pure consciousness. Maharishi explains that in this phenomenon,

> the image of the flower travels to the retina of the eye and reaches the mind. The image of the flower impressed on the mind gives the experience of the flower. The result is that the mind, as it receives the impression of the flower, is overshadowed by that impression. The mind's essential nature is obscured; the image of the flower remains impressed on it. The observer, or the mind, is as though lost in the experience.

With the regular experience of transcending, however, pure consciousness rises more and more into the nature of the mind, and ordinary waking consciousness becomes transformed. And when cosmic consciousness is fully established, Maharishi explains,

> the impression will be there, because the flower will be seen, but it will be like a line on water. It is drawn, it is seen, and yet simultaneously erased. This is how the fullness of the state of Being [pure consciousness] is maintained, and at the same time the outside, objective experience is maintained.

Maharishi emphasizes that it is not by thinking about pure consciousness, or by trying to maintain a mood or intellectual idea of pure consciousness in the mind while experiencing objects, that the mind achieves this level of development. It is only by the simple process of transcending and directly experiencing pure consciousness that its nature spontaneously rises in the mind, giving us the experience of pure, unbounded bliss at the same time as we are enjoying the exterior world to the maximum. Maharishi also makes the point that cosmic consciousness is not a state of withdrawal from life. Far from it, because the experience of pure consciousness increases the conscious capacity of the mind, and therefore our experience of objects becomes deeper, richer, and more substantial.

Maharishi describes how the continuing refinement of the neurophysiology results in two more advanced states of consciousness. In the sixth state of consciousness, called refined or glorified cosmic consciousness, perception becomes so refined as to appreciate the finest values of every object of perception along with unbounded pure consciousness.

Whereas in cosmic consciousness the knower realizes his essential nature as pure consciousness, the sixth state involves the refinement of the more expressed values of the knower—the mechanisms of perception. One begins to perceive the subtler values of the object of perception. It is as if the qualities of pure consciousness, firmly established at the deepest level of subjectivity, begin to spill out into the objective world of what we see and hear.

The seventh state of consciousness, traditionally referred to as unity consciousness, is the pinnacle of human development—complete enlightenment. In the state of unity, inner and outer realities are seen in terms of their most universal and unbounded nature—the Self. One knows pure consciousness to be the underlying reality not only of one's own subjective nature, but of every object of perception in the objective world. One comprehends change and non-change, the two fundamental aspects of life, simultaneously and sees that they are nothing other than the expression of unbounded pure consciousness—the wholeness of the unified field of natural law moving within itself. Maharishi comments, "The enlightened man, while beholding and acting in the whole of diversified creation, does not fall from his steadfast Unity of life, with which his mind is saturated and which remains indelibly fused in his vision."

Maharishi emphasizes that the growth toward higher states of consciousness occurs naturally through the practice of Transcendental Meditation. Higher states are not experienced as something strange or bizarre; rather, we experience them as completely natural states of awareness.

From my own research, I am convinced that as scientists we need to explore more deeply the anatomy of consciousness and the patterns of development of higher states of consciousness. We have set our sights too low. By seeking knowledge of human life and health with a focus on the physiology of matter alone, we have raised our eyes only as far as the foothills. As the mountaineer Maurice Herzog said as he neared the peak of Annapurna,

> There was something unusual in the way I saw my companion and everything around us...all sense of exertion was gone, as though there were no longer any gravity. This diaphanous landscape, this quintessence of purity—these were not the mountains I knew: they were the mountains of my dreams.
>
> When the clouds clear—that will be when we avail ourselves of the knowledge of both the finest mechanics of natural law, and their immense practical applications for human life. This is nothing less than the complete understanding of health and human physiology—and when we know this, then we will know the high peaks in all their splendor.

CHAPTER 2

Quantifying the Patterns of Transcendence

Learning to transcend is the first prerequisite for studying the anatomy of consciousness. To transcend means to go beyond. In the case of Transcendental Meditation it means that the conscious mind goes beyond the limitations it experiences in the ordinary states of waking, dreaming, and sleep. In Transcendental Meditation, one transcends the ordinary excited levels of thinking—the boundaries of the mind—and experiences deeper, quieter, and more powerful levels of the thinking process. Eventually, even thinking is left behind, and the mind experiences the self-referral dynamics of the unbounded field of pure, transcendental consciousness.

Transcending is essential to Transcendental Meditation. One can read many elaborate, often obscure descriptions of various forms of meditation. However, Maharishi makes it clear that the single, inflexible criterion for any true form of meditation is that it enables the mind to settle into a state of deep silence while remaining awake—that is, to experience its basis in transcendental consciousness. Maharishi's restoration of the fundamental principle of transcending is fortunate for all human beings, and also for science.

We might ask, "If transcendental consciousness is such a desirable state, why has it been virtually ignored and disregarded by advanced Western society?" The principal reason is that a reliable, verifiable technology for experiencing transcendental consciousness has not been available. Without an effective technology to systematically refine mental activity, transcendental consciousness became merely an esoteric topic of discussion.

Imagine what would happen if the world somehow returned to a primitive state, but with all the machinery of modern technology left intact. After a few generations, without scientists or technicians to explain how a modern power station worked, the equipment would break down and become useless. Untrained in its use, people would eventually ignore it, and the knowledge it represented would become misinterpreted or simply disappear. Even a manual on how to repair the equipment would seem useless, or possibly even mystical, if one couldn't understand its technical jargon.

This analogy is not so different from what has transpired over millennia in many countries. Once there did exist very lively and effective traditions of gaining higher states of consciousness. Yet in India, as well as in other countries, they remained vital only as long as the people conscientiously followed the correct meditation procedures. Some traditions of knowledge were disrupted because of upheavals in the social or political structure. Historically, invasion and subsequent domination by an outside culture weakened the inner integrity of native culture and traditions. In some countries, particularly India and China, meditation was taught only to a select few monks; the common people, whose focus was on the daily routine of living, were not instucted. There may have been thousands of reasons for the decline of knowledge, but the overall result was that fewer and fewer people within the parent traditions continued to achieve and maintain higher states of consciousness.

Because only an isolated few were experiencing higher states, there was no common ground on which such experiences could be understood. The vast majority of people who were not living in higher states began doubting the entire method. Since it was inaccessible to them and to most other people, why should they believe the experience of a few older seers who lived apart from the mainstream of society? What was once regarded as the highest level of knowledge, the pinnacle of truth and practical achievement, came to be regarded as mystical and impractical.

With Maharishi's revival of the correct methodology, it is now possible to systematically and repeatedly experience transcendental consciousness. Besides providing enormous practical benefits for the individual, this methodology has made it possible for us to experientially and experimentally explore the relationship between the physiology of consciousness and the physiology of matter in the development toward higher states of consciousness.

Research on Consciousness

In this new paradigm, we can assume that while consciousness is the basis of matter, consciousness requires the material physiology to support its activity. In order for the physiology of consciousness to act and develop, it needs the physiology of matter. Therefore, whenever the mind experiences transcendental consciousness—a subjective state of completely expanded awareness—something measurable must show up in the body at the same time.

Physiological recordings cannot tell us what the experience of transcendence feels like. But the patterns they display are a way of tracing the fingerprint that the state of transcendental consciousness leaves upon the body, both during and after the experience. By studying a wide range of physiological and biochemical parameters, we are perceiving the patterns in this fingerprint in increasingly fine detail. These patterns are one means we have of understanding and quantifying the fundamental patterns of nature's intelligence lively at the basis of human experience, and seeing how they affect the whole physiology and individual health.

Maharishi's introduction of the Transcendental Meditation technique to the West in the late 1950s made systematic research on consciousness possible for the first time.

Because the technique is taught in a systematic and reliable way, the researcher is assured that all subjects are using the same procedure. And because instruction is available practically everywhere in the world, subjects are readily available. From their first day of TM practice, individuals frequently report the effortless experience of a state of inner silence, inner wakefulness, and inner peace. The degree of clarity of the experience of transcendental consciousness may vary considerably, but everyone has a taste of it because of the inherent naturalness and effectiveness of the technique. Such experiences became the focal point for my initial research.

I began research in 1967 as a graduate student at the UCLA Physiology Department and Brain Research Institute. At the time I conducted the research, I had no idea of the impact it would have. Since then, there have been over 675 sceintific studies conducted at more than 300 institute in more than 30 countries on the effects of the Transcendental Meditation program and over 380 of those studies are published in peer-reviewed journals. Peer-review methods insure that scientists of good qualifications and competence have thoroughly evaluated the research.

The Physiological Patterns of Transcendental Consciousness

A major finding that physiological studies on the TM technique have revealed is the unique state of "restful alertness" that subjects experience: the body settles down to a state of deep rest and relaxation, while the mind is fully awake and alert. During TM, for example, subjects show a decrease in heart rate, respiration rate, oxygen consumption, and plasma cortisol and lactate levels, and an increase in skin resistance and EEG (electroencephalographic) coherence.

Many early studies took a general approach, comparing the average magnitude of a particular variable (such as respiration rate) during experimental and control periods. There was no attempt to isolate and characterize specific periods in which subjects were experiencing transcendental consciousness.

In later years there was an attempt to more carefully identify the subjective experience of transcendental consciousness, and to characterize this subjective experience by specific objective markers. The Transcendental Meditation technique is dynamic, having both an inward phase and an outward phase; during the 20 or so minutes of TM practice, subjects go in and out of transcendental consciousness many times.

Subjects report that in the inward phase, their mental activity settles down to quieter levels until they eventually transcend all mental activity, yet remain awake in the experience of transcendental consciousness. In the outward phase, they emerge from transcendental consciousness, and more excited states of mental activity gradually reappear, preparing the way to begin the inward phase again.

The degree of clarity of the experience of transcendental consciousness (subjectively reported) varies greatly, as do the frequency and duration of each of these inward and outward phases. Subjects who are overly tired before practicing Transcendental Meditation report having short periods of drowsiness or even sleep during meditation. Throughout the the practice of the TM technique, there is often a mixture of the active waking state, drowsiness, sleep, relaxation, quiet waking state, and the experience of transcendental consciousness.

The mixture of states that occurs during TM practice is a direct consequence not only of the initial condition of the individual's nervous system, but also of the dynamics of the procedure itself. The deep rest during the technique allows the system to "normalize" itself—that is, to remove any functional or structural abnormalities and regain its normal healthy patterns of functioning. Everyone is familiar with this principle: when we rest during a cold or illness, the body's internal system spontaneously attempts to remove any foreign invaders and to heal itself.

The same principle applies to the practice of TM. As the mind becomes less active during TM, the body settles down and becomes restfully alert. Its internal systems automatically begin to remove any deep-seated stresses or abnormalities. This normalization process causes a stir of activity. The mind shifts out of transcendental consciousness, becoming more active as it returns to a more excited state, or becoming less active to the point of drowsiness or even sleep.

What is perhaps most significant about these and other physiological studies is that they have shown us that transcending is not exclusively the province of Indian or even Eastern physiology. The machinery and patterns of transcending are part of the genetic endowment of the human nervous system. Whether we use it or not, transcending is an inherent ability. In fact, Western literature is filled with descriptions of states of restful alertness that are strikingly similar to the patterns of transcendental consciousness, as are the personal records of people in many different cultures throughout the ages. Although one rarely reads of anyone who regularly experienced this state via the use of a systematic technique, many have experienced it at least once or more in their lives.

Alfred Lord Tennyson vividly describes a beautiful transcendental experience:

> ..all at once, as it were out of the intensity of the consciousness of individuality, individuality itself seemed to dissolve and fade away into boundless being, and this not a confused state but the clearest of the clear, the surest of the sure, utterly beyond words—where death was an almost laughable impossibility—the loss of personality (if so it were) seemed no extinction, but the only true self. I am ashamed of my feeble description. Have I not said the state is utterly beyond

Patterns of the Brain

One of the most important and useful developments in brain research on TM has come through the application of a measurement called brain wave coherence. Brain wave coherence measures the orderliness of the electrical activity of the brain and helps answer the question, "Is the activity of one area of the brain correlated with the activity of another?" Brain wave coherence measurements during the TM technique helped further distinguish the pattern of physiological changes during TM from those seen in sleep or drowsiness; in both sleep and drowsiness any consistent, strong coherence in the alpha and theta bands is lost. Further, in TM subjects clearer experience of transcending was associated with higher levels of brain wave coherence.

One study compared three types of meditation practices, classified according to their brain wave or EEG signatures. The first type is called focused attention meditation. These techniques entail voluntary and sustained attention on a chosen word, phrase, or object and are characterized by EEG in higher frequency bands called beta and gamma.

The second type is called open monitoring meditation. These techniques involve non-reactive monitoring of the moment-to-moment content of experience, and the most popular of these is known as mindfulness. The EEG is characterized in general by a slower theta wave activity. For example, EEG recordings from Zen meditation, Vipassana meditation, and Sahaja Yoga, "open monitoring" styles of meditation, show an increase in slower theta waves in the frontal and central areas of the brain.

The third type is called automatic self-transcending meditation. The primary technique here is the Transcendental Meditation technique, which involves effortless transcending (or going beyond) the normal experience of life to experience a more unbounded state of self-awareness free from all thoughts or feelings, other than the sound value of a specific word or mantra. The EEG changes during the Transcendental Meditation technique primarily involve an increase in the alpha wave activity, especially brain wave coherence. This increase has been found not only during the practice but also in TM meditators during activity, indicating a higher level of integration of brain functioning.

Brain imaging technique also show striking differences among the three different types of meditation. Research on focused attention meditation in which subjects were practicing Tibetan Buddhist loving-kindness-compassion meditation, has found significant activity in areas associated with sensory processing, emotions, and attention. Researchers using brain imaging studies on the second type of meditation, Buddhist mindfulness meditation, find increases in cortical thickness in certain areas. Brain imaging during TM shows a decrease in activity of areas concerned with sensory processing and an increase in the activity of the frontal areas concerned with executive functions.

The conclusion from this and other studies is that different meditation techniques produce different results. My own research has been focused on the Transcendental Meditation technique because I feel it is the easiest and most effective technique for achieving higher states of consciousness. I believe we now have the means for realizing the full range of human development—the state of enlightenment. Enlightenment is not abstract or mystical—on the contrary, it is very practical, involving a holistic pattern of systematic refinement in neurophysiological functioning.

CHAPTER 3

The Chemistry of Consciousness

India is the land of meditation, a land of yogis and saints. Various forms of meditation are such an intimate part of the tradition and culture that practically everyone is familiar with it. When I once asked a bright young group of medical students in South India whether they might be interested in meditation, especially if I could show strict scientific research on its benefits for learning, health, and longevity, very few expressed interest. I wasn't sure whether this was because of the long-held misunderstanding that pervades India about the mystical and impractical nature of meditation, or if it just came from the lack of a rational explanation for how something so familiar and common could have such good and scientifically verifiable effects.

I then asked the students how many might be interested if I were to offer a new pill, developed in our Western laboratories, which could improve their memory and have beneficial effects on their health and longevity. Virtually all the students raised their hands; they were more than willing to take this new pill. Granted, these were medical students, yet medical students are more aware than the public of the shortcomings and side effects of pills. Why, then, were they so eager to take a pill rather than meditate?

Finally I asked, what if I could demonstrate that during meditation a new chemical was produced, and that this chemical was identical to the pill I was offering them (i.e., it markedly improved mental and physical functioning) would they then be interested in meditation? This time the students all raised their hands enthusiastically. As long as I could explain the mechanics of meditation in terms of pills and chemicals, then there was no prejudice, no misconception. Everyone takes pills for instant relief. We understand how they work, and we want even better ones. They are part of the classical paradigm. Meditation, however, is part of a new paradigm of consciousness. Only when meditation is explained in the mechanical terms of the old classical paradigm, does it become more readily acceptable.

Actually what I was offering to the students was not merely a fanciful idea. Today, laboratories around the world are attempting to isolate a single chemical that could help explain the physiological and psychological changes seen during the Transcendental Meditation program—a single chemical that would link the physiology of consciousness with the physiology of matter.

Ojas and Soma

Through the years Maharishi has referred many times to two substances frequently mentioned in the Vedic texts. These substances, known as *ojas* and *soma*, are considered to be the body's natural mediators of perfect health, longevity, and the experience of higher states of consciousness. Let's consider soma first.

Maharishi explains that in the Vedic literature, the word soma has several meanings. In its broadest sense, soma refers to a basic tendency of nature that holds the universe together, the flow of the underlying self-interacting dynamics of consciousness.

Soma also refers to a chemical produced in the body as a result of achieving a stress-free state of consciousness. As Maharishi describes:

> ... a normally functioning nervous system, free from stress and strain and any abnormality, produces a chemical called soma.... If there are no restrictions, no inhibitions, then awareness is unbounded, and when this unbounded awareness is maintained spontaneously at all times, then the nervous system is functioning normally.... Now the by-product of a normally functioning digestive system is soma. Soma is that which helps all the fundamentals of individual life to develop themselves so that the totality of individual consciousness may rise above boundaries, and have an unbounded status.

In this context, soma is both the product of neurophysiological refinement and the very substance that enables the development of full mental and physical potential. The principle that every state of consciousness is supported by a physiological state is interpreted here to mean that soma is the key biochemical that supports the experience of transcendental consciousness and eventually enlightenment. This "elixir of longevity" is distilled not in a pharmaceutical lab, but through the process of the inner development of consciousness. Soma is a product of the body's natural pharmacy, created by a nervous system functioning in higher states of consciousness.

Certain texts in the Vedic literature that pertain specifically to health further elaborate the definition of soma. In these, "soma" refers specifically to the first definition—an abstract dynamical principle of consciousness that is capable of unifying diversity in nature. For the second definition (a unique chemical in the body responsible for ideal health and longevity), the term ojas is used. Ojas and soma are intimately related. They represent the same unifying principle in nature. However, soma is that unmanifest principle expressed in consciousness; ojas is its manifest expression as the finest possible level of matter. We could say that ojas is the first material, biochemical expression of soma in the physiology of matter, which is the basis of all the succeeding layers of matter in the body—cells, tissues, organs, etc.

Ojas is considered a biochemical that establishes balance between the physiology of consciousness and the physiology of matter. Because it is located at the junction point between consciousness and matter, ojas is described as being like "a lamp at the door," illuminating both the inner field of consciousness and the outer field of matter.

One last definition of soma: the Vedic literature also refers to a particular plant or herb of this name, traditionally used during special ceremonies. Among the many medicinal properties attributed to this plant is the ability to increase longevity.

Searching for the Biochemical Basis of Transcendental Consciousness

For several years, researchers have been trying to better understand the neurophysiological and biochemical mechanisms of Transcendental Meditation. They have, in fact, been involved in a search for ojas and soma. A number of research groups have found changes in various biochemicals and hormone levels, such as a reduction in plasma cortisol or stress hormone. The search for the biochemical basis of transcending is one of the most exciting frontiers in research on consciousness.

This research can be greatly accelerated by an understanding of deeper levels of the physiology. Biochemical pathways in the body are often controlled by enzymes which are, in turn, produced by genes. Genes are packets of information in our DNA which ultimately control all biochemical and physiological processes.

One of the most promising directions of research on the biochemical effects of the TM technique is on gene expression. Two studies have shown changes in the expression of different genes as a result of the practice of TM. In one study it was found that TM increases the production of an enzyme called telomerase, which has been correlated with increased longevity. In another study, over 70 genes were found to be changed in practitioners of TM as compared to control groups. A more thorough analysis of changes in gene expression as a result of Transcendental Meditation could help us discover not only the biochemical nature of soma or ojas, but also the mechanics of how TM produces so many beneficial changes is health. This research will further help establish a bridge between the divergent understandings of the physiology of consciousness and the physiology of matter.

We now think of the body not as a localized bundle of cells and tissues, but as one mind-body network of intelligence. The primary means for the integration of this mind-body network is through biochemical communicators such as hormones, neurotransmitters, and neuropeptides. Discoveries about the action of neuropeptides in influencing behavior have given us a far more detailed understanding of how this mind-body network functions. The finding that many different types of cells throughout the body can both send and receive messages via the neuropeptides has enriched these discoveries. As more and more biochemical messengers are discovered, the picture will become increasingly more comprehensive.

We will be able to objectively discern the fine details of the mind-body network. Further, as a result of this integrated research, we will finally have a complete system of knowledge, understandable to scientist and layperson alike, of the underlying biochemical mechanics of the development of higher states of consciousness.

CHAPTER 4

Consciousness and Health

A number of years ago I had an appointment to meet with a fellow researcher at a prestigious New York hospital. When I arrived, I was invited to wait in the head cardiologist's office. As I entered the room I noticed a live video monitor connected to the main operating room, on which I could hear and see an open-heart surgery taking place. A very angry surgeon was interrogating the cardiologist about his diagnosis. The patient's chest lay open, but the surgeon could find nothing wrong with the heart. The cardiologist maintained that all the preoperative tests had shown that one of the heart valves was malfunctioning, but the surgeon could see that this was simply not so. Everything was perfectly normal. The discussion went on with the patient, his chest open, lying unconscious on the table between them. Finally, the surgeon declared, "Well, now that I'm in here, I'm going to replace the valve anyway!"

At that point I had lived most of my life with great confidence in modern medicine. How naive was I? Should the cardiologist or the surgeon be blamed for the unnecessary operation? I knew enough about biomedical equipment to know how difficult it was be to interpret certain results. I also knew that what I had witnessed was not exactly an everyday occurrence. Yet I am appalled at a system that is so complex and out of our grasp as patients that we can become victims not only of disease, but also of its treatment. Even with the most sophisticated tools and years of medical training, not only is it possible, it is not uncommon for doctors and even specialists to incorrectly diagnose and treat a critical condition.

Iatrogenic disease, the disorders caused by modern medicine, are widespread and of grave concern. Just entering a hospital can be a risky act. The problem is the enormous emphasis we put on treating the symptoms of disease and how little we do to prevent the disease arising.

The Damaging Effects of Stress

In the 14th century, an epidemic of plague wiped out one-third of Europe's population in less than one hundred years. The epidemic of the modern world is stress. Heart disease is the number one stress-related disorder and is by far the greatest health problem of the Western world. It causes more adult deaths than all other diseases combined. While there are clearly genetic factors (and others such as diet and smoking) that make some individuals more predisposed to heart disease, it is stress that ultimately precipitates the fatal attack.

Stress is a hidden killer; it is all around us and continually affects us. There are numerous factors known to increase stress, including the death of a loved one, loss of a job, financial difficulties, divorce, lack of sleep, and tense work situations. One stress seems to attract another, and the cumulative action of multiple stresses has even more damaging effects on the body. Stress disrupts the flow of intelligence in our physiology of consciousness; it manifests as structural or functional abnormalities deposited in the system and eventually results in disease in our physiology of matter.

Many diseases such as ulcers, insomnia, and headaches are thought to be due in part, or at least complicated by, an inappropriate or prolonged response to multiple-stress situations. Each day, whether caused by a traffic jam, a boss's remark, or a quarrel at home, the harmful effects of the stress response are having an impact on our health and longevity. It is no wonder that the harmful effects of stress are so strongly linked to heart disease.

Heart attacks and strokes were at one time considered a by-product of aging. Scientists had observed that blood vessels became narrow and less flexible with aging. Also, the buildup of hard, fatty deposits inside the artery walls increases year by year in many people, leading to high blood pressure, heart attacks, and strokes. The majority of Americans show these conditions as they age. However, more and more studies suggest that this process is neither normal nor inevitable. It is a product of our stressful civilization and of our inability to deal with the increasingly fast pace of life.

There are some simple cultures, removed from the stresses of Western life, which have almost no heart disease. This is the good news. We don't all have to be subjected to the newest operations of modern medicine. If nature did not mean for the heart and arteries to degenerate with age, then heart conditions should be preventable and reversible if caught in time. Research indicates that this is indeed possible.

Stress Management

Rest and relaxation can help relieve some symptoms of cardiovascular disease. Patients asked by their doctors to go to the hospital often temporarily recover from the adverse symptoms of cardiovascular disease just because they are forced to rest. Yet it is almost impossible to have prolonged rest. Therefore, the only practical approach is to try to periodically quiet down and relax our overactive systems. That's why stress management programs have become very popular. There are many programs, and almost all of them work on the principle of relaxation. If stress arouses the physiology, then the way to counteract stress is to "de-arouse" the physiology—to relax.

Rest and relaxation can be antidotes to stress. Sleep itself removes stress. But usually the rest and relaxation of normal sleep is not enough, and sometimes we are actually too stressed to sleep. Stress management programs offer some small help by periodically reducing our level of stress. Occasional relaxation during the day can counter a few of the adverse effects of stress and fatigue. However, most stress management programs offer only superficial rest and relaxation. We need a far deeper rest to remove the deep-seated stresses that accumulate in our lives. These deep-seated stresses create subtle imbalances in our physiology, which, when they accumulate, lead to disease.

Where does stress enter the body? It enters through consciousness. Before a stressful experience affects our body it must usually first pass through our senses and emotions to the central nervous system. The brain acts as a filtering device that sorts which experiences are to be recorded and responded to. Filtering enables us to cope with all the external demands of the environment. If this coping ability is somehow hampered or overburdened, then stresses freely accumulate and tax our entire body.

How do we increase our coping ability? According to Maharishi, the key to managing stress is to transcend and evolve to higher states of consciousness. If we want to remove darkness from a room, we don't try to manage the darkness. Darkness is merely the absence of light. By turning on a light switch we automatically remove the darkness. Likewise, the way to remove stress is to go beyond it, to evolve. The process of transcending in Transcendental Meditation takes the mind to the state of pure consciousness, which is entirely free from stress.

Unlike sleep or relaxation, in which the body is resting but the mind is either unconscious or dull, transcendental consciousness is a state in which the body is resting deeply while the mind is filled with unbounded awareness and bliss. It is a type of rest in which the nervous system becomes highly integrated and coherent. This restful alertness is not only the most powerful antidote to stress, but the most effective way to remove deep-rooted stresses already deposited in our nervous system.

Further, the regular experience of transcending acquaints the nervous system, little by little, with a state in which silence and activity can coexist. As we develop toward cosmic consciousness, we can be immersed in rigorous activity, yet not lose the experience of unbounded awareness. We are no longer overshadowed or exhausted by stressful experiences and therefore are better able to cope with environmental stress. As described earlier, experiences no longer leave deep impressions etched in our nervous system; the impression is more like a line on water. Many studies on the Transcendental Meditation program show precisely this effect. When subjects practicing TM were given stressful stimuli, they were physiologically able to recover far more quickly than non-meditating controls. The meditators also showed many long-term physiological and biochemical changes, indicating improved neurophysiological functioning.

The Transcendental Meditation program enables individuals to evolve to healthier states. The TM technique has often been referred to as a "stress management" technique. It is indeed a powerful technique for the management of stress—but that is merely one of its positive side effects. The primary purpose of the technique is "evolution management," the development of higher states of consciousness, so that we can begin to use the full potential of the nervous system and live in perfect health.

Improvements in Health

Approximately $25 million in federal aid from the National Institutes of Health have funded well-controlled studies that clearly show the beneficial effects of the TM program on high blood pressure and heart disease. Studies have also demonstrated the positive effects of the TM program on reducing cholesterol levels and decreasing tobacco and alcohol use.

The most significant study on TM and cardiovascular health was conducted at the Medical College of Wisconsin in Milwaukee. Measured over five years, 201 middle-aged and elderly African Americans, with an average age of 58, were randomly assigned to either a health education group or a TM group. The TM group had a reduced risk of 47% in heart attacks, strokes, and deaths as compared to the non-TM group. This is a remarkable finding, far better than any drug currently available.

Several studies have clearly shown that the TM technique reduces rates of hospitalization and doctor visits as compared to control groups. For example, health care costs related to heart disease were 87% lower than the norm for the TM group. The rate of hospital admission for the TM group was 63% lower than the norm for nonsurgical medical procedures, and 71.5% lower for surgery. The rate of doctor visits was 58.8% lower. These differences were not due to meditators intentionally avoiding medical care—for example, health care usage rates for obstetrics were similar in both groups.

One of the most significant findings was that the decrease in health care utilization was even more striking for older people. Meditators over 40 years of age showed health care costs that were, on average, 75% lower than those for nonmeditators in the same age group. This would seem to indicate that the beneficial effects of the TM program actually increase as we get older.

These studies have extremely important implications for our own health care system as well as those of other nations. They give us the answer as to how we can immediately and dramatically reduce health care costs.

CHAPTER 5

The Search for Longevity

I remember one of the first lectures I ever heard Maharishi give in the mid-1960s in Los Angeles. In that talk he described how TM could increase longevity. These words had an enormous impact on both my personal life and my professional career. They inspired me to enter the field of physiology. They were the basis for my doctoral thesis and for subsequent research on transcendental consciousness and its effects on the aging process. They gave me a different perspective from which to view the body. I began to see the physiology of consciousness and the physiology of matter as one integrated network, which, when fully enlivened, has enormous potential benefit for health and longevity.

Aging and Prolonging Life

Trillions of organisms grow and die every second. Innumerable physical structures are created and destroyed. Yet the element of nonchange is implicit in biological organisms.

From the broad perspective of biological evolution—in the perpetuation of a species—the whole purpose of life indeed seems to be directed toward prolonging life.

For most organisms, prolonging life means the continuity of their DNA. Their entire lives are designed around the single function of reproduction. Perhaps there is no better example of this phenomenon than in the life of the Pacific Northwest salmon. Hatched in inland streams, baby salmon migrate to the sea. Once they reach maturity they undergo an epic journey to return to their original spawning grounds and ensure the "longevity" of their species.

The ability of certain living creatures to maintain the existence of their species over millions of years is a remarkable feat of nature. Even man's greatest monuments, such as the pyramids of Egypt, created by highly developed civilizations to record and glorify their power, have slowly eroded, and continue to crumble away into fine grains of sand. It is inevitable that over time the order of a physical system will tend to dissipate, to mix with other elements of the environment. Yet many of the organisms that live in the cracks of decaying pyramids and in the surrounding sand existed as species long before the civilizations that built those monuments were born. These organisms will continue to exist for centuries to come. Perhaps they will find their way onto a spacecraft someday and be carried to other hospitable planets where they will outlive even the earth itself.

One of the very great achievements of this century has been the discovery of the DNA molecules structured within the core of all living organisms. This source of all biological information, which forms the main constituent of our genes and chromosomes, is the universal code from which the enormous variety of life forms, from bacteria to man, have evolved. DNA's most extraordinary property is its capacity to adapt, regenerate, and self-perpetuate. Because of this capacity, the information contained in DNA is literally millions and millions of years old, yet shows no sign of aging.

The ability of living systems to maintain stability and continuity amidst great upheavals speaks for the intelligence that underlies and organizes their existence. If that intelligence is powerful enough to allow for the longevity of a species and within certain single-cell organisms such as bacteria (which divide continuously and thus never die), is it possible for longevity to be structured within an individual human being?

In an age in which great scientific discoveries are natural, even common, there are leading researchers in the field of aging who feel that extending longevity is entirely possible. All our mental and physical functions are constantly improving to some optimal level until the age of twenty or thirty, and then it all changes. We begin to age. Why?

Why Do We Age?

Two basic theories of aging are prevalent today: aging is due either to a predetermined genetic program or "clock," or to the accumulation of errors and the gradual breakdown of the system.

According to the genetic clock theory, the damage or disorders seen in older organisms are not the result of a random or accidental process, but rather of a specific genetic program. For example, the process of aging is similar to other stages of development and is controlled by a specific set of "aging genes." When the aging genes are activated, they regulate the gradual breakdown of the organism. Just as other developmental stages are orchestrated by the information in DNA, so too is aging.

According to the error theory, aging occurs because the organism is unable to properly repair errors that accumulate over time. The precise cause of this accumulation of errors is a subject of great debate among researchers. As a result, error theory itself has led to many different theories of aging.

Balance: The Inner Wisdom of the Body

We have developed a very impatient and combative attitude in our problem-solving approach in the field of health and aging. Our sense of long-term planning, whether it applies to our own individual lives or to our overall environment, is very limited. We tend to favor immediate solutions: if you overeat and feel pain, take Alka-Seltzer; if you overwork and get a headache, take an aspirin; if you get too stressed and can't sleep, take Valium; if you want to live longer, take some new wonder drug.

It's a very strange philosophy of life—one which puts us always at odds with the natural tendencies of our physiology. We feel we can do whatever we want and then take a drug or have an operation to correct the consequences.

For example, we know that heart disease is preventable, but we continue to do the very things that aggravate the condition, almost as if we are challenging nature. Technology is our savior; if our arteries become clogged, we can replace them with new ones. This same careless "godlike" attitude has also crept into the field of gerontology, the study of aging. Gerontologists can be very bold, feeling that it's only a matter of time before they create a wonder drug that will defy death and ensure longevity.

When I listen to the claims of gerontologists seeking to unlock the gates of longevity, I am genuinely interested. Because of my own scientific training, I appreciate their logic, and I have no question about their sincerity or belief that life extension is possible, for I share this belief. But what I do object to is their purely mechanistic attitude and approach.

The body is a hierarchical network of interlocking feedback systems. The primary function of these systems is to maintain balance and internal stability. They resist every attempt to manipulate them by chemical means. If you increase someone's levels of a certain hormone by injecting it into him, his body's intricate feedback systems will resist the outside change—they will compensate by increasing or decreasing production of the hormone, to keep it at its predetermined set point. Of course, if the drug is powerful enough and taken in a sufficient dosage, it acts like an atomic bomb on the system. The body can't defend itself and is overwhelmed. Some of its reactions may be beneficial, especially in relieving acute symptoms. However, many of its other reactions may result in devastating side effects.

How, then, can top gerontologists believe that life extension is merely a matter of artificially increasing a hormone, taking some new wonder drug, or manipulating a few genes? With numerous theories about the aging process, each offering a new potion, it becomes quite difficult to know which program really does influence longevity.

In an age of genetic engineering there is an enormous potential for both oversight and undersight. As we gain deeper knowledge into the laws of nature and develop the technology to tamper with these laws, our responsibility for proper and holistic judgment increases beyond any expectation.

We must remember that the body possesses its own inner intelligence. For any effective longevity program to be safe and complete, it must use and enliven this inner wisdom of the body.

The Effects of the Transcendental Meditation Program on the Aging Process

Studies on aging conducted at Duke University have correlated seven factors with aspects of aging and longevity. These are, in order of significance: cardiovascular disease, work satisfaction, cigarette smoking, physical function, happiness rating, self-health rating, and performance IQ.

Studies on people who regularly practice the Transcendental Meditation technique show improvements in all seven factors. Cardiovascular disease risk factors such as high blood pressure and high cholesterol levels improve. Job satisfaction improves. Cigarette smoking and alcohol consumption decrease. Physical functions (such as motor reactions, respiratory and circulatory functions, and sensory performance) improve. Meditators show increased happiness ratings, contentment, self-regard, and self-actualization, and decreased anxiety and neuroticism. Increased happiness is further demonstrated by the significant improvement in hospitalized patients suffering from severe depression. These findings arc also of interest in light of a study conducted at Harvard University, which clearly establishes that better mental health is associated with longevity. Meditators also show improvements in self-health ratings and on IQ tests designed to measure fluid intelligence.

Other studies have focused directly on measuring biological markers of the aging process in elderly TM subjects.

It was found that long-term TM meditators had significantly younger biological ages than short-term meditators, controls, and norms for the general population, and that the strength of this effect was related to the length of practice of the TM technique. Long-term practitioners of the TM technique and its advanced programs had biological ages that were on average twelve years younger than their chronological ages.

A well-controlled study conducted at Harvard University showed that Transcendental Meditation improved health, longevity, and cognitive and behavioral flexibility in elderly individuals as compared to controls doing mindfulness and relaxation programs. The most striking finding was that in addition to reversing age related decline, TM appeared to directly enhance longevity: all members of the TM group were still alive three years after the program began, in contrast with an average 76.6% survival rate for the other groups and a 62.5% survival rate for residents in the same facilities who were not included in the study.

The results of these studies, supported by the large number of other physiological studies, strongly indicate that the Transcendental Meditation program slows and even reverses the aging process.

Promoting Longevity in Change

Maharishi emphasizes that at its most profound level, the level of the unified field of natural law, the physiology of con-

sciousness is immortal. It is in the mechanism of manifesta-
tion, the transformation from the physiology of consciousness to physiology of matter, that the seeds of aging are sown.

Another example of this phenomenon in physiology is
seen when even one or a few abnormalities in the sequence
of nucleotides in DNA can result in fatal diseases—for example, sickle cell anemia. "Evolution," Maharishi comments,
"is certainly a system of change, but the system of change
does not have to be dragging to life, because the change also
is structured in nonchange." Change in reality is only an ex-
citation of the nonchanging unified field. In the process of
evolution, the field of nonchange appears as change—the un-
changing nature of the unified field is hidden from view by
all the changing diversity of creation.

According to Maharishi, ignorance—forgetting our ability to experience and be in tune with the immortal nature
of our physiology of consciousness—is the reason for aging.
Maharishi states, "Enlightenment is just a matter of awak-
ening. Nothing happens in the state of enlightenment other
than we gain the awareness of unboundedness, the awareness of immortality." It is only a process of remembering our
inner nature, of waking up to our full unbounded potential.

For every state of consciousness, there is a corresponding state in the physiology. If consciousness is established on
the level of perfect balance, then the physiology will reflect
that quality. The orderly sequential flow of awareness will be
accompanied by a corresponding orderly flow of physiologi-

cal functioning. If there is some disruption or imbalance in the expression of the dynamics of consciousness, then that becomes manifest on the gross level of the physiology in the process of aging.

Maharishi explains that "when the awareness has no memory of the unbounded, then this is the aging process." He connects the process of aging with the inability to live in harmony with all the laws of nature: "Aging is directly associated with natural law, and if there is a violation of even a few of the laws of nature, then aging will keep on breathing."

In higher states of consciousness, the underlying unity of life, the unified field of the laws of nature, is the permanent reality of our lives. The sequential unfoldment of the laws of nature is perfectly orderly and balanced in this state. All the programs developed by Maharishi, especially the Transcendental Meditation program, are designed to enable each individual to naturally and effortlessly achieve higher states, live in tune with the total potential of nature, and therefore not violate any laws of nature. Thus in the Vedic tradition, the simplest and most practical formula for disallowing aging is to become enlightened.

CHAPTER 6

The Week War Ended

His excellency will see you now."

The voice startled me, so intent was I on trying to hear any sound from the outside world. Even artillery fire would be muffled where we were, I decided. This was my first visit to a dictator's bunker. Looking around when we first arrived, I was surprised to find it decorated with comfortable overstuffed chairs and plush carpeting. One hardly noticed that the curtains had no windows behind them, not even slits.

"If you'll step this way," the guard murmured. I trailed behind the small group that rose to follow him. We were a delegation of three American scientists visiting Central America on a peace mission. We had come to Nicaragua in response to a plea that had appeared in the press from the citizens of a town devastated by the violence of a brutal civil war. The people were calling for any national or international agency to bring relief: "Anyone who can help, please help." Maharishi wanted to respond immediately. We arrived in this small nation more or less unannounced, but after several phone calls we were granted an audience with its head of state.

Peace was a good calling-card just then. After years of using the country as his own private reserve, El Presidente's rule was rapidly crumbling. The rebel forces, labeled as Communists by the government and as liberators by themselves, were gathering outside the capital. The final assault was expected at any time. Many thought it was overdue.

When we entered a large office, the face that greeted us was instantly recognizable from the six o'clock news back home as the country's president.

"If you don't mind," the president gestured toward chairs near his desk. Then he returned to the phone conversation we had interrupted. He was a large, imposing man, impeccably dressed in a three-piece silk suit.

"Don't worry, Tom," he said into the phone, "the situation is completely under control. There's a little trouble, it's nothing we can't handle. We are still very interested in making the deal." I gathered that he was talking, not to a field commander, but to an old friend in the United States. Years ago the president had made connections at Harvard Business School. Now he apparently assumed that he could still run his country on the basis of business as usual.

I marveled at the unreality of his view. In October 1978, the decay of power was in the very air of Nicaragua. The day before, we had visited its parliamentary chambers. Terrorists had sprayed the building with machine-gun fire. I looked up and noticed hundreds of bullet holes in the elaborately decorated ceiling. On the way to the bunker, we had seen armed soldiers in combat fatigues on every corner.

When his phone call was over, the president asked us to begin. There was a brief pause. None of us had ever been in quite this position before. The first to speak was Dr. Lawrence Domash, a Princeton trained physicist who headed our group. "We are American scientists who have come to brief you," he began, "on a new technology that can bring peace to your country."

The dictator nodded. He did not seem perturbed, or for that matter surprised.

"We are a special group formed to bring about world peace," Dr. Domash said. "Approximately 150 of this group are living in the hotel there"—he gestured in the direction where a window would have faced our hotel, if a window had been there—"and at this moment we are using this new technology to calm hostilities within your nation."

"What exactly are you doing?" the man asked.

"We are meditating. That is the core of this technology. It is the first technology of its kind, based entirely upon consciousness. But I would like to lay out our proposal for you in full. May I?" He began to bring out some papers.

"Please," the president said politely.

We brought out a copy of that week's local newspaper and held it up for him to see. On the front page was a picture of a large group of young men, most of them under thirty, all dressed in coats and ties, all smiling.

"As you can see from the coverage," Dr. Domash pointed to the story, "we announced our intention on the day of our arrival to prove that we could bring peace to your nation." He handed over more recent issues of the same paper. "Our formal research results will not be forthcoming for several months, but as you can see from these accounts, your press has in fact reported a drop-off in war-related incidents since our arrival. This is an article commenting on the sudden lull in hostilities that has begun."

I wondered if "war" was the word the president would have chosen to describe current events, but it passed without comment.

"Because this technology cools down negative tendencies of all kinds," Dr. Domash continued, "we also expect from our past experience that you will see a decrease in crime, particularly here in the capital, and extending to other parts of the country. Also, hospital admissions and road accidents should have decreased in the past week. Relations with neighboring countries could suddenly improve. All of these benefits will continue, we feel certain, so long as the meditators maintain their presence here."

The man leafed through the papers, then silently handed them back.

"Presently," Dr. Domash said, "similar lulls in hostility and even cease-fires are being created in southern Africa, the Middle East, and Southeast Asia. Sometime during this month or next, in order to demonstrate conclusively that this technology works, we hope to see a halt in all major conflicts around the world."

Since the dictator continued to regard us with polite interest, we began to relax. Two days earlier, we had boarded a jet in Miami, scheduled to stop in several Central and South American countries. Many of them were military "hot spots." The meditators involved in our peace efforts had preceded us into the region by about two weeks. The majority were based nearby, but smaller groups had quietly taken positions in the neighboring countries.

Because we felt convinced that we were on the verge of changing mankind's whole concept of political power, everyone was committed to bringing our project to the attention of national leaders, no matter what their reactions might be. We felt confident in the influence we could create, even though we had never before confronted a ruling head of state with our aims.

The Meissner Effect

Dr. Domash continued, "Essentially we are taking advantage of well-known principles that apply in physics. But we are applying them to a new area. In physics, Newton's third law of thermodynamics holds that if you decrease the temperature of a physical system, then the system increases in orderliness. Ice, for example, is a more orderly and stable form of H_2O than water.

"Moreover, if you have an impurity dissolved in the water, such as salt, the water will spontaneously purify itself as it freezes. In a glass of salt water, as the temperature is lowered toward the freezing point, a layer of salt is deposited in the bottom, and you are left with a mass of ice above it that is pure H_2O.

"A group of meditators can produce orderliness in the same way. Violence, hostility, and the collapse of law and order are disorderly expressions of consciousness in a society. If you can cool down the collective level of awareness, then collective consciousness can restore itself to orderliness, just as the water can rid itself of the salt and form a stable, orderly structure of ice crystals."

I watched the dictator carefully while Dr. Domash talked. It was obvious that he caught on, at least partially, to what was being presented. This in itself was an achievement. We knew that from the viewpoint of conventional politics, we had come from the moon. We wanted to convey that what we actually represented was an entirely new perspective.

The future of the nation did not lie with El Presidente or with the rebels. Each looked upon the other as an implacable enemy, but in fact they had one common enemy—their own chaotic consciousness.

Dr. Domash went on, "A more profound example of the principle of reducing activity and thus increasing orderliness and purity is seen in the phenomena of superfluidity and superconductivity. If the temperature of liquid helium is decreased to a few degrees above absolute zero, an extraordinary phase transition occurs, producing a unique fourth state of matter different from the gaseous, liquid, or solid states—known as the superfluid state. In this superfluid state, helium can escape through glass containers; it becomes as if unbounded. Its resistance to flow is zero, and its capacity to conduct heat is infinite.

"If the temperature of a metal, such as lead, is reduced to a few degrees above absolute zero, a similar type of phase transition occurs, resulting in the phenomenon of superconductivity. One of the unique properties of a superconductor is its property of invincibility, known as the Meissner Effect. When a magnetic field is brought near an ordinary conductor of electricity, it penetrates into the interior of the conductor and disturbs the flow of electrons inside. On the other hand, when a magnetic field is brought near a superconductor, the superconductor produces a magnetic field that precisely cancels the intruding field. The result is that no external magnetic field can penetrate into the superconductive region. This same principle applies to a nation. By utilizing the Transcendental Meditation technique and its advanced programs, we can create a highly coherent state in the collective consciousness such that no damaging outside force can penetrate."

In our delegation was Dr. David Orme-Johnson, one of the first researchers to study the collective effects of the Transcendental Meditation technique and its advanced programs. He was the next to talk to the president. Dr. Orme-Johnson opened up a map of Central America with certain regions marked in red. "As you can see, we have placed a core group of meditators here to create the desired cooling effect on hostilities. Smaller groups have been positioned in neighboring countries. They are not large enough to create an effect on their own, but they strengthen it from the outside.

"We are proposing to leave these groups in place for the next two months," Dr. Orme-Johnson explained, "so that the government will have time, if it is satisfied with the results, to assume responsibility for continuing the project.

"In each country we need to train meditators, enough so that the effect will persist. In the beginning, that would amount to instructing a large number of people, up to one percent of the population. We would supply the teachers; all we ask is that you reimburse us for our expenses.

"However, the numbers can be drastically reduced. The meditators are now practicing a much more powerful advanced program. We could begin to teach this technique within the next year, and then only a core group, of less than three hundred people, could maintain peace in your country."

This would be the stickiest point, we knew. Although he looked very tired and under tremendous strain, the dictator had listened to us. Now we expected him to act. It often happened, when we presented our program, that government officials showed tremendous enthusiasm while we were physically with them. We expected to hear from them afterwards, but there would be only silence. The gap between their situation and the solution we were presenting was too great for them to bridge alone.

Transcendental Meditation is regarded as a means for self-development. From the start, however, Maharishi taught that it had much wider implications. At a time when Westerners were just absorbing the idea that their own consciousness could be developed individually, Maharishi posed an incisive analysis of unrest on a social scale:

"Where there is disagreement and dissension in families or in a group of friends, the disharmony seems to occur only in a small area. Individuals do not realize that through ill-feeling, malice, bad behavior, harsh words, and suffering, they are contributing to the disruption and destruction of the peace of the world."

Maharishi places the individual at the center of the world, proposing that the unit of world unrest is each individual; therefore, the unit of world peace must also be the same:

"The problem of world peace can be solved," Maharishi explains, "only by solving the problem of the individual's peace, and the problem of the individual's peace can only be solved by creating in him a state of happiness."

Maharishi presented this simple logic in 1963 in his first book, *Science of Being and Art of Living*. He had been stating it to audiences from the first day when he walked out from the Himalayas and began to teach TM. Whatever the public thought he was accomplishing, Maharishi measured his success by one standard—bringing peace to every single person in the world. In the early years, his strategy had been utterly direct: he intended to teach Transcendental Meditation to as many people as possible in every country on earth. By raising their standard of happiness, he would raise the happiness of mankind. It was a strategy of pure numbers.

By the early 1970s, however, his strategy had become much broader. He had successfully "multiplied" himself, as he liked to put it, by training a large, dedicated corps of Transcendental Meditation teachers. But even with many teachers, it was obvious that getting the whole world to meditate would take too long. Even though he saw the decrease of stress and negativity in the consciousness of meditators, there was obviously growing tension in the world as a whole.

The Maharishi Effect

The progress toward world peace needed to take a quantum leap, and in 1974 it did just that. By that time, Transcendental Meditation was being practiced on a wide enough scale that some cities in the United States had one percent or more of their populations meditating. Examining the statistics from four Midwestern college towns, the original "one percent cities," psychologist Garland Landrith observed a decrease of crime in those areas once they reached the one percent threshold. The scientists appropriately named this phenomenon the "Maharishi Effect." A later analysis confirmed that a sudden drop in crime rate occurred as soon as any city crossed the one percent mark. The decrease held firm, on average, for at least six years.

Scientists theorized that some type of phase transition must be occurring in the general awareness of society. As soon as a core number of meditators created orderliness in the collective consciousness of society, orderliness increased everywhere. The decrease in crime was really just a ripple on the surface. The real action took place at a subtler level.

Maharishi called the subtler level "collective consciousness," the sum of the consciousnesses of all the people in the society. In the past, collective consciousness has never been studied in a serious scientific manner, because it could be neither isolated nor experimentally experienced. The most sophisticated sociological theories give at best a vague description of a social field as an interlocking network of social and behavioral interactions within specific economic and environmental conditions.

The Vedic tradition removes misconceptions and ambiguities, presenting the concept of collective consciousness from a more complete perspective. We have not only an individual physiology, but a collective physiology—the physiology of society—in which each of us is like one cell in a large superorganism. The physiology of society has its own physiology of consciousness and its own physiology of matter. Its physiology of consciousness encompasses the collective consciousness of all the individuals. Its physiology of matter encompasses all material activities of all individuals.

In the case of the one percent studies, the physiology of society under consideration was that of a community or city. But the effect did not have a theoretical limit. If it could influence positive trends in society, then it might also be applicable to a nation or even the world. On the world scale, the equivalent of crime is terrorism and war. Therefore, if the meditators exerted a coherent enough influence, they should accomplish something amazing—they should put an end to war.

The Extended Maharishi Effect

In 1976 Maharishi introduced an even more powerful technology called the TM-Sidhi program. The Transcendental Meditation technique allows your mind to settle down to the source of thought and experience pure consciousness—a state of restful alertness. The TM-Sidhi program trains you to think and act from this most silent and powerful level of the mind. The TM-Sidhi program was brought to light by Maharishi from the Yoga Sutras of Patanjali, from the ancient Vedic tradition. The TM-Sidhi program is designed to accelerate the growth of creativity, learning ability, physical health, and psychological well-being that TM technique practitioners report. Maharishi explained that the TM-Sidhi program develops the ability of the individual to act from the unified field of all the laws of nature. He predicted that on this basis, a comparatively small number of people—the square root of one percent of a population—practicing this program in groups should be sufficient to produce measurable effects on the various quality-of-life indices in any society.

The rationale for this prediction came from discussions with leading physicists concerning coherent effects seen in physical systems, particularly in the laser, which exhibits a state which is known in physics as superradiance.

This was the effect we were testing during this world peace project in many parts of the world. We were closest to the square root of one percent in Lebanon and Nicaragua, and there the hostilities suddenly dropped off—some observers said it was as if a switch had been pulled. This was the first large-scale experiment testing the "square root of one percent" effect, which became known as the Extended Maharishi Effect.

The purpose of our presentation to the Central American dictator, however, was not to propose a scientific experiment, but to offer to stop war in his country and create a thriving and peaceful society. Unfortunately, it was clear that we were not getting through. The huge gulf between the dictator's world and the one we were sketching was obvious to all of us in the room. At a certain point, after we had been talking for perhaps an hour, a phone call came, and he excused himself to take it.

I leaned over to Dr. Orme-Johnson. "What can we do?" I whispered.

"I think we're losing him."

"Do anything," he said. "Give him your slide show."

Indeed that was about all the ammunition we had left. When the president turned to face us, I introduced myself as a physiologist.

"I realize," I began, "that what we've told you seems very abstract." The expression on his face indicated how right I was.

"There is another side to meditation that is not abstract at all," I said as I set up the projector. "I have been conducting research on TM and stress. What I have found will interest you."

Lights dimmed. I flashed a slide on the wall that illustrated the decline of blood lactate during Transcendental Meditation. The next slide showed EEG measurements, emphasizing the alpha-wave peaks of meditators. To me, these are rather technical, but for the first time the man looked fascinated.

"Show me more of that, if you would."

There was a lot more to show—all of the many findings on Transcendental Meditation. I explained the EEG changes in detail because these results establish the high degree of coherence that is established within the individual.

As slides of more and more findings appeared on the wall, I made the point that these were the first modern proofs that the age-old practice of meditation had scientific validity. I pointed out, as tactfully as possible, that if Americans could benefit from reduced stress through meditation, then certainly his own people could.

"Stress is within the individual," I said, "but it is also out there in the environment. War and civil unrest are expressions of collective stress, and what we are offering is a way to reduce it."

"Yes, yes," he responded eagerly.

"If one person can use this meditation to reach a level of consciousness where he does not suffer from stress, then could an entire nation not benefit even more?"

It was the closest we dared come to saying, "Look, you and this country are in deep trouble. Let us help."

The man sat thoughtfully. Then he stood and congratulated us on our presentation. He seemed genuinely impressed and completely persuaded. He warmly shook my hand as we left, promising that he would be in touch soon. It even occurred to me that he might become the first government leader in history to support a nationwide program to create coherence in collective consciousness. We waited for his call, and then, because of the high cost of maintaining many groups of advanced TM experts in these trouble spots all over the world, the group had to leave. It was not entirely surprising to hear that within months he had been violently deposed and rebel leaders were now firmly in power.

The World Peace Project

Flying over the aqua waters of the Caribbean on the way to Central America, we had considered the risks we were running. Maharishi's peace experts were deliberately stepping into places that could erupt into full-scale violence at any time. Some of the hot spots in the world that year included Iran, Lebanon, Nicaragua, and Southern Rhodesia (now Zimbabwe).

Every location was crackling with tension, especially in Iran. At one point, the hotel in Tehran where the meditators were based appeared to be under siege. Mobs opposed to the Shah were pillaging the city, concentrating on the sections where foreigners resided.

The job of the scientists was to explain the principles of the Extended Maharishi Effect to the heads of state in each country. Transcendental Meditation had undergone scientific scrutiny for more than a decade. By the time our delegation met with the various government leaders, there was a core of research findings that strongly validated our claims about the scientific mechanisms involved in creating world peace.

The research also gave us credentials in the countries we visited and helped explain the otherwise baffling phenomenon that one observer called "an outbreak of peace." Looking back now, I cannot help but admire the meditators' commitment and dedication to creating world peace. I later read in the newspaper a first-hand account of the Iran peace project by Jon Levy of Ithaca, New York:

> The forty of us were volunteers—freedom fighters, if you will—only the freedom we were fighting for was the freedom to be happy and to live without fear, and the fighting was done in a seated position with eyes closed. Teachers of the Transcendental Meditation program experienced in the TM-Sidhi program were being sent to Iran by His Holiness Maharishi Mahesh Yogi, the founder of the TM program, to change the chaos to harmony and the disorder to orderliness....
>
> Seeing the degree of chaos that prevailed made the task seem almost impossible. True, I had seen a profound transformation in my own life and in others I instructed in the TM technique. And I had seen studies which show the environmental value of a small percentage of people gaining that level of "least excitation of consciousness" through the TM program: reduced crime rates, lower admissions to hospitals, less violence, and increased quality of life.
>
> But this was something else. This was tanks and machine guns on one side and fanaticism and Molotov cocktails on the other. When we arrived in Isfahan (a smaller city about 200 miles south of Tehran).... we were welcomed by the sound of the hotel closest to ours being blown up and twelve of the city's banks being set aflame.
>
> And so there remained nothing to do but to get on with it. Tanks rumbled by our hotel as we settled into meditation and the TM-Sidhi program (an advanced series of techniques designed to develop perfect coordination between mind and body). As the first day turned into night, we began to sense a growing feeling of separateness from the turbulence going on around us. By the second day we were feeling very at ease, despite our external environment, and by the third day there was no denying the profound experience of "invincibility" which permeated everyone on

the project. There was no fear, no anxiety, only a strong undercurrent of silence and peace.

On the fourth day the value we had been experiencing overflowed into our environment. It could be easily noticed, even by those not in any way connected with our project. The sun came out, children returned to their play in the streets, the troops were not so much in evidence, the shops reopened, the cacophony of human and vehicular sounds which enunciate a healthy marketplace was, for the first time since we arrived, heard throughout the city....

Peace prevailed throughout the land. Nobody knew why. Almost nobody, anyway. As our inner experiences became even more profound, the orderliness around us reflected that value. The tanks disappeared. The bazaars reopened. Schools throughout the country, which had been closed by the violence, again echoed with the cheerful voices of Iranian children....

Perhaps the strongest single bit of evidence of our success occurred on "Army Day," an event which honors the national militia with parades and display of military hardware. It was thought opponents of ... the Shah would seize the opportunity with a bloody confrontation.

Instead, the people threw flowers at the passing troops, and no shots were fired anywhere in Iran that day.

Peace could be felt in every country the meditators visited. In Rhodesia (now Zimbabwe), the rate of war deaths fell from an average of 16 per day to 3, starting the week the meditators arrived. In the countryside, 2,000 insurrectionists changed sides and enabled the transitional government to hold peaceful elections. Black leader Bishop Abel Muzorewa, flanked by guerrillas who had turned in their weapons, told an assembly, "Peace has at last taken hold of our war-torn society." The BBC's Iranian correspondent reported an inexplicable calm in the atmosphere after months of extreme chaos.

By the last weeks of December 1978, the World Peace Project was over. After maintaining some 1,400 meditators in hotels for an extended period, sometimes as long as four months, in groups ranging from 30 to 400 strong, financing had become an issue. We could not carry the burden of continuing the project without assistance. The various groups in Iran, Rhodesia, Nicaragua, and other countries were forced to pull out. There was some concern that if our influence made the cessation of hostilities possible, then our departure might easily tip the balance back the other way.

This appeared to happen in several places. War deaths in Rhodesia sprang from 3 per day back up to 16, the old level, as soon as the meditators left. A truce had begun in Lebanon in October, just as the meditation group responsible for that area landed in Israel. The truce lasted three months, making it one of the longest of the bloody civil war.

When the group in Israel broke up in January, the truce collapsed, and war casualties immediately went up to pre-October levels.

In Iran the situation was potentially so explosive that removing the meditators at the end of four months had to be orchestrated like a military withdrawal. Maharishi told us that the peacemaking effect would collapse almost immediately after our groups left the country. Therefore, it was imperative to take them all home on the same day. Otherwise, an upsurge of violence could engulf any small group left behind.

We had groups scattered around the country, in Tehran, Isfahan, Tabriz, and Shiraz. To move them all out on the same day required that the groups in the south fly across the Persian Gulf at the same time that the northern and central groups flew to the Tehran airport. Then both contingents departed simultaneously for America on synchronized flights from Tehran and Saudi Arabia. Maharishi was emphatic about this maneuver, and we quickly understood why. Four days after our evacuation, mobs forced the Shah to flee Iran, and a few days later, amidst near chaos, the Ayatollah Khomeini returned from exile to assume power.

It is important to make it clear that we did not choose sides in any country we visited. Our personal opinions of the politics of the Shah or the Central American dictator (or the opinion of them held by the press) were not at issue. In all the volatile regions of the world, regimes rise and fall; ideologies follow each other in quick succession. Our concern was to create coherence in the collective consciousness. Maharishi explains that any government is only an "innocent mirror" of the collective consciousness of the people it governs. If collective consciousness is stressed and turbulent, the actions of the government will reflect that. In the current situation, creating coherence in collective consciousness through the Extended Maharishi Effect could not only end violence and suffering as quickly as possible, but it would transform any government, whatever its ideology, to be just and good.

The international news at the end of our project spoke to us in a way that no one else in the world could understand. On November 18, the International Herald Tribune quoted President Carter on his opinions about US-Soviet relations: "I think that in recent weeks there has been an alleviation of tension between us, and I would like to see it continue." The president also commented that he did not know any concrete reason for the improvement.

Amid such scattered reports, including peace initiatives from the Soviet Union and the ratification of a historic treaty between China and Japan, a small item was carried in several American papers on November 30:

> Despite border clashes, cold wars, internal turmoil, and lagging peace treaty negotiations, no nations are actively engaged in open warfare at the moment—a historic rarity.

That was the week war ended. This item was not data that scientists could use, but we remember it anyway.

There was, however, ample statistical data on the effects of the World Peace Project. Obviously, the effect of peace was not permanent. The national governments we contacted did not choose to back the project with their own funds, although many officials had enthusiastically responded in private. A few of them even started TM. The scientists' data had confirmed that during the period of Maharishi's World Peace

Project, a statistically significant reduction in hostility had taken place around the world—one which could not be accounted for either by chance or by previous political trends. They created coherence in the collective consciousness of society as a whole. These new technologies had demonstrated the power of consciousness to create world peace.

CHAPTER 7

The World Is My Family

The sun glittered off the cascading water of the Vltava River as I walked across the Charles Bridge in Prague. I couldn't help but think of the awe and wonder a young village boy must have felt on his first journey to this magnificent city. The remarkable towers of the famous St. Vitus' Cathedral sit high on the hill overlooking the ancient city, known as the "City of a Hundred Spires," one of Europe's finest jewels.

I was here at perhaps the most historic moment in the city's long history, a turning point in the balance of world power. Only a few months earlier, Prague had peacefully overthrown its communist rule, and now its new president was in Washington addressing the US Congress. I got back to my hotel room just in time to see the live broadcast. It was a brilliant speech, leaving no question about the importance of the unbelievable turn of events that had transpired in 1989.

President Havel boldly said to millions of people listening worldwide, "Consciousness precedes physical being, and not the other way around, as the Marxists claim....Without a global revolution in the sphere of human consciousness, nothing will change for better in the sphere of our being as humans." These words echoed the feelings of the people throughout all of Eastern Europe and much of the Soviet Union.

What had happened in Czechoslovakia was happening everywhere. With the dismantling of the Berlin Wall, the terrible fear and tension that existed among the superpowers had rapidly begun to dissolve. Clearly, this time will be regarded as one of the greatest moments in the history of the world—when the Cold War ended and a new era of international cooperation began. It was the precursor to other events, including the end of Soviet communism and the breakup of the Soviet Union itself, that were even more astonishing, even miraculous. The march of world events starting from 1989 produced a complete phase transition.

How and why did this powerful momentum of change in the world take place in 1989 and since? Was it due to negotiations or peace treaties? There are many explanations. Numerous books have been written and will continue to be written on the subject. Researchers have estimated that there have been approximately 9,000 peace treaties over the last three thousand years, with an average life span of just eight years.

The World Peace Project of 1978 produced the first real data that revealed the power of consciousness to calm down violence in different countries. The scientific research on the effects of these groups and on several major peace projects conducted in subsequent years gives clear verification that it was the technology of consciousness that changed the world and established world peace in 1989.

Experimental Confirmation of the Maharishi Effect in the Middle East

One of the most striking demonstrations of reducing international conflict was conducted in Israel in the summer of 1983. The International Peace Project was initiated by the Institute for Research on Consciousness and Human Development at Harvard University. The study was supported in part through a grant from the Fund for Higher Education in New York.

This was a prospective study, in which certain specific results were predicted before its actual implementation. The study aimed to gather together in Jerusalem 200 people, the square root of one percent of the population of Israel, to collectively practice the Transcendental Meditation technique and its advanced programs. Because many of the participants had professional responsibilities, the actual number of participants varied from week to week, reaching 200 during one two-week period and on several weekends. This constantly varying pattern actually enabled a more careful statistical analysis of the Extended Maharishi Effect.

Results of the study clearly demonstrated the effect: when the number of participants went up, there was a significant decrease in reported war deaths in Lebanon, a decrease in the intensity of the Lebanon war (as measured by news content analysis), a decrease in fires and automobile accidents in both Jerusalem and in Israel as a whole, and an increase in the Israeli stock market. Using a statistical procedure known as time series analysis, a clear relationship was determined between the overall quality of life in Jerusalem, Israel, and Lebanon (as measured by a composite index of many different variables) and the number of TM-Sidhi participants.

The study was submitted to one of the most prestigious and conservative journals in the field, the *Journal of Conflict Resolution*, edited at Yale University. It took more than three years before it was finally published. In any paradigm shift, there is often a battle between old and new ideas. It is difficult for researchers to accept a new hypothesis, especially when it so clearly conflicts with their existing ideas. This is precisely what occurred in the publication of this study.

Creating World Peace

The most ambitious and widely publicized demonstration of the effect of group practice of the Transcendental Meditation technique and its advanced programs on world peace took place in Fairfield, Iowa, home of Maharishi University of Management, for three weeks at the end of 1983. This marked the first time the Maharishi Effect was tested on a global scale. The demonstration was an assembly called "A Taste of Utopia." It was announced as a global sociological experiment and was the first time in world history that more than 7,000 people—the square root of one percent of the world's population at that time—gathered to collectively practice their TM and TM-Sidhi program.

Dr. John Hagelin and coworkers created one of the last demonstration projects in 1993 in Washington, DC. An independent panel of more than twenty sociologists, criminologists, and members of the Washington, DC. government and police department advised on the study design and reviewed the analysis of the findings. Over 4,000 people gathered in Washington to participate in a peace assembly. The experimental design employed Box-Jenkins time series transfer function analysis. The results showed that as the group size increased, there was a highly significant decrease in violent crime from predicted levels, reaching a 16% reduction when the group was largest.

To date, there are more than 50 studies on the Maharishi Effect and the Extended Maharishi Effect. The scope of these studies ranges from the effects on cities and states, to those produced by a group in one country on the national life of that country, on neighboring countries, on international conflicts, and on the world as a whole. Taken together, the research provides us with experimental evidence of an effective technology to create peace in the world.

In the post-Cold War era, every country must secure its own inner integrity by increasing coherence in the collective consciousness of its people. This will create not only strong

TRANSCENDENTAL MEDITATION

and prosperous nations, but a harmonious family of nations, like a beautiful mosaic made up of many patterns. With this will come a new style of international relations, in which the attitude of every nation toward every other nation will be, as the expression in the Vedic literature states, *Vasudhaiva kutumbakam*—"The world is my family."

Maharishi explains that governments are an "innocent mirror" of collective consciousness. Government leaders—however much they as individuals may want to act for the good of the nation—can only express in their thinking and behavior the level of coherence in collective consciousness. They cannot act for positivity unless collective consciousness is positive. If collective consciousness is full of turbulence and negativity, then the actions of political leaders will only express that.

Ironically, this has sometimes produced a "catch-22" situation, in which the leaders of the very countries that most badly need coherence may actually be aware of, and even interested in adopting, Maharishi's programs. However, they have been prevented from acting in favor of complete positivity by the very turbulence in collective consciousness that they seek to amend.

One of the most interesting studies also helps explain why these many studies on the Maharishi Effect were not acted upon by governments. This was a doctoral thesis done at Harvard University and later published in the *Journal of Social Behavior and Personality* by Dr. Carla Brown. This paper examined how five different groups of elite members of the Middle East policy community—peer reviewers, newspaper reporters, Congress-people, non-governmental experts, and US diplomats—assessed the International Peace Project on the Maharishi Effect conducted in the Middle East.

What is particularly interesting about Dr. Brown's research is how the different experts in Washington reacted to this study. It is, without question, a controversial study since it challenges the current paradigm. So it comes as no surprise that the different groups in Washington who were given this study generally did not believe its results. Dr. Brown, however, found that over half of each group reviewing the research rejected it immediately without even examining its scientific merit. This, she explains, has to do with their prejudice against scientific research that does not conform to their own beliefs and not even to the unusual nature of this particular study. She did note that there were a few who did assess the scientific quality independent of their own belief, philosophies and practices.

Our government leaders, despite their best intentions, cannot eliminate problems. Thus the responsibility for establishing these groups lies with the people of the nation.

Maharishi's Master Plan to Create Heaven on Earth

Maharishi's goal was to establish groups of 7,000 to stabilize the coherence in world consciousness, prevent jerks and jolts in the current phase transition to an ideal world, alleviate the remaining areas of violence, and make world peace permanent.

In Maharishi's view, however, world peace was not enough. Peace is not just the absence of war. For Maharishi, establishing permanent, irreversible world peace was only the beginning. The effect of having several permanent groups of 7,000, he said many times, will be not only world peace, but an improvement in the quality of life for everyone on earth.

Through the technologies of consciousness Maharishi has brought to light from the Vedic literature, many age-old aspirations can be realized in this generation. In place of fear, hatred, disease, misery, and poverty, Maharishi has offered a very real way to create unlimited peace and fulfillment.

Maharishi had suggested that the groups of 7,000 could be created in education institutions where the students' nervous systems would be cultured to radiate peace and unfold their full mental potential. By including TM in our educational system, we automatically provide every individual with the knowledge and experience of how to develop higher states of consciousness and, as a byproduct, create world peace. Maharishi describes the outcome of such an education as "the fruit of all knowledge"—a mistake-free life lived spontaneously in accord with all the laws of nature.

Chapter 8

Education for Enlightenment

The meeting that took place in 1971 at the University of Massachusetts was all over the media. Two men were on stage, looking like beings from different worlds: Buckminster Fuller, his white hair clipped short, and wearing a dark suit and black rimmed eyeglasses, was seated at a conference table with a microphone in front of him; his demeanor was serious. Maharishi Mahesh Yogi was long-haired, in a simple garment of white silk, with monk's beads and a flower garland. Sitting cross-legged on an elegant sofa, Maharishi held a single red rose; his face was gently amused.

When Fuller spoke he addressed the contrast in their appearance, explaining that he had long ago decided to endeavor to look like a "second-rate bank clerk," becoming "invisible to others" in order to further his highest goals. "It is just in clothing," he added, "that we (Maharishi and I) are different."

What Buckminster Fuller and Maharishi Mahesh Yogi had in common was a burning interest in furthering the greater good of mankind.

Fuller went on to say, "I am sure what makes Maharishi beloved and understood, is that he has manifest love. You cannot meet with Maharishi without instantly recognizing his integrity. You look into his eyes and there it is."

At this, Maharishi remarked laughingly, "Often they may be closed."

Fuller continued,

> That Maharishi is spontaneously engaging the love, understanding, and support of the young is the most important manifestation we can have of that beautiful integrity. So, I'd like to say that it is great news that young America has its arms open for the truth and love and tenderness—compassion. And the only way in which we can know the truth is through our mind. Our young world first manifest great abhorrence for the non-truth, for the superficial misleading information of our customs. Now that young world is gone beyond just being dismayed, and being disapproving of the non-truth, but is demonstrating in this wave of inspiration by Maharishi, demonstrating its yearning, its determination for humanity to survive on our planet. Very deep forces are operative here, the forces of the great intellect of the universe itself, and this is news. It is not easy to report in the newspapers this kind of news, but this is the news.

With his characteristic delight in wordplay, Maharishi responded: "This is the vision of 'fuller' life for the world."

This historic exchange between Maharishi and Buckminster Fuller was part of a series of conferences that took place in the early 1970s, during which Maharishi unfolded a new and holistic approach to education called the Science of Creative Intelligence. At this symposium, Maharishi clearly distinguished between the two fundamental methodologies of gaining knowledge:

The Western scientific approach to knowledge is based on the non-variability of the objective means of observation. The Eastern approach to knowledge is based on the non-variability of the subjective means of observation. Speaking for the East, we know there is a level of consciousness called *"ritam bhara pragyan,"* which is non-variable in its nature; and therefore, on that level, the knowledge of an object never changes, remaining authentic and truly scientific for all time. Western science has continued to contribute to the advancement of civilization because good minds in the West have persistently applied the objective methodology of gaining knowledge, whereas Eastern civilization has not continued to contribute to the advancement of civilization because good minds in the East have not persistently applied the subjective methodology of gaining knowledge. Rig Veda proclaims that knowledge is structured in consciousness. Now the teaching of Transcendental Meditation—in the structure of the Science of Creative Intelligence—enriches the knowledge of the West and revives the knowledge of the East and will give the benefit of both methodologies to every man in the world. The Science of Creative Intelligence is the glorious meeting ground for the Eastern and Western ideals of gaining knowledge. All men everywhere will enjoy the highest ideal of life in fullness of all glories, material and spiritual.

The Science of Creative Intelligence was the beginning of Maharishi's development of an ideal system of education, and over the next 30 years, he re-enlivened the full value of the ancient Vedic knowledge in his Vedic Science and Technology of Consciousness.

Maharishi's Vedic Science and Technology of Consciousness

Maharishi's Vedic Science and Technology of Consciousness is the study of the intelligence of nature and its accessibility to man in the simplest state of his own awareness. It explains that intelligence has two aspects, expressed and unexpressed, manifest and unmanifest. The expressed level is clearly seen in the orderly behavior of the laws of nature, and in man's ability to understand these laws. The unexpressed level is in the field of pure consciousness, which we experience when we transcend the finest levels of our mind.

It is precisely because the Vedic method of gaining knowledge depends upon a fully developed nervous system, that its main field of inquiry, the field of pure consciousness— the experience of inner Self —became inaccessible when the procedures to gain higher states of consciousness were no longer readily available. Over the long course of history the experience of pure consciousness faded in daily life and the knowledge of the Veda became greatly misunderstood and misinterpreted. The situation was further complicated when the Vedic texts were written down and eventually translated into other languages. What remained was not true knowledge based on experience, but its outward and superficial expression. It took Maharishi over 50 years to revive the depth and scope of this remarkable knowledge, much of which is now incorporated into the curriculum of the different schools and universities he established throughout the world.

Maharishi University of Management

It was during the symposium with Buckminster Fuller that Maharishi founded Maharishi International University in the US, later renamed Maharishi University of Management (MUM). The idea for the University was Dr. Nat Goldhaber's inspiration, and I was privileged to serve as its first President.

Located in Fairfield, Iowa, MUM is fully accredited to the doctoral level and offers an undergraduate liberal arts curriculum, along with specialized graduate programs. What makes the University unique is its Consciousness-Based approach to education, through which students can acquire a high level of academic achievement while developing their inner and outer potential with regular practice of Transcendental Meditation.

The educational program at MUM stands as an ideal model for all other universities. It has been evaluated by numerous leading educators, who always remark upon the high quality of the students, the excellence of the faculty, and the extraordinary sense of harmony and progress evident throughout the university. Commencement speakers at MUM graduation include CNN chief political correspondent Candy Crowley in 2012, Senator Tom Harkin in 2013, Jim Carrey in 2014, and Yukio Hatoyama, the former Prime Minister of Japan in 2015.

The University has established an elementary and secondary school, Maharishi School of the Age of Enlightenment, graduating ten times the national average of National Merit Scholar Finalists, with 95% of its graduates accepted to four-year colleges. Maharishi School students in grades 10 through 12 continually score in the top 1% of the nation on standardized educational tests.

In state speech competitions, Mahrishi School students have won more awards than any other school in the state's history. In sports, they have won 16 boy's state tennis championships, more than any other school during the same time period.

Throughout the years, Maharishi's Transcendental Meditation technique and educational ideals have been introduced to students in a number of schools in the US and other countries. The results have been dramatic, with reductions in violence, and improvements in test scores, as well as more positive student and teacher interactions. In a study conducted by researchers at the University of Michigan, the meditating children showed significantly more positive emotions, positive mood states, and greater emotional adaptability than their non-meditating peers. Meditating children also had higher self-esteem, more positive well-being, improved management of stress and interpersonal skills, and less verbal aggression, anxiety, and loneliness. These improvements have been repeated in many other schools where TM was introduced. Teachers comment that classes become more settled, there is greater mutual respect, and students are more eager to learn.

Researchers have also shown that the Transcendental Meditation technique could be learned and successfully practiced by children with attention deficit-hyperactivity disorder (ADHD) and that it had the potential to reduce anxiety and stress-related ADHD symptoms within three months. They noted that TM produced significant changes in brain functioning, opposite to that of ADHD, and which was correlated with the improved behavior and performance in the students.

Experience changes the brain. The experience of transcending, as we have seen, produces many benefits. By including TM within our educational system, we provide the neurophysiological mechanisms to reduce stress, improve academic performance, and unfold the full creative potential of each student.

Numerous studies have shown the many psychological benefits in students and adults practicing TM, such as reduced anxiety and depression, and increased energy level, self-esteem, tolerance, creativity, and intelligence. In an excellent comparative study, researchers clearly show that the changes in the anxiety levels of TM subjects are significantly different from those seen in control subjects practicing different relaxation techniques.

In addition, there are studies which show improvements in self development and self-actualization, as measured by tests on the research and theories of Abraham Maslow. This is particularly interesting since Maslow's description of self-actualization has a number of similarities to Maharishi's description of the growth of higher states of consciousness. In an analysis of 42 studies, researchers showed that the effects of Maharishi's Transcendental Meditation technique on self-actualization were markedly greater than that of other forms of meditation and relaxation.

These psychological improvements have important applications in other settings. For example, studies have reported that when TM is introduced into businesses, there is greater job satisfaction, a reduction in stress, improvements in health and employee development, improved performance, and better relations with coworkers and supervisors. In addition, studies have reported improvements in leadership, management, and organizational development. A number of studies in various prisions have shown that the TM technique produces long-term beneficial psychological changes, with a markedly reduced rate of recidivism, or return to prison.

The very wide range of physiological and psychological studies shows how important it is to introduce TM in every area of life. The expereince of transcending during TM cultures a new style of neurophysiological functioning, which enables anyone to achieve the highest level of human development, enlightenment.

Traditionally, the process of gaining enlightenment is referred to as a procedure of becoming more and more fully awake inside—awake to the inner dynamics of consciousness. The poet Thoreau recognized the value of being fully awake and beautifully summarizes the importance of this state:

> Moral reform is the effort to throw off sleep. Why is it that men give so poor an account of their day if they have not been slumbering? Had they not been overcome with drowsiness they would have performed something. The millions are awake enough for physical labor; but one in a million is awake enough for effective intellectual exertion, only one in a hundred million for a poetic or divine life. To be awake is to be alive. I have never yet met a man who was quite awake. How could I have looked him in the face?

The David Lynch Foundation

One of the main organizations responsible for the introduction of TM to students is the David Lynch Foundation. A good example of its success can be seen in three schools in the San Francisco area, the Visitacion Valley Middle School, the Everett Middle School, and John O'Connell High School, which offer the TM technique as part of their regular program. Research shows that teenagers who practice TM in these programs show improved academic performance and test scores, increased self-esteem and greater happiness, decreased anger, anxiety, depression and fatigue, and reduced symptoms of learning disorders. In one school system there was an 86% reduction in suspensions, as well as a 40% reduction in psychological distress, and a 65% decrease in violent conflict over a two-year period.,

The David Lynch Foundation is supported by numerous cultural and creative leaders, such as Paul McCartney, Katie Perry, Ellen DeGeneres, Dr. Mehmet Oz, Russell Brand, Laura Dern, Moby, Martin Scorsese, and Jerry Seinfeld, and others. The Foundation has brought Transcendental Meditation to over half a million school children in the United States, Brazil, Peru, Bolivia, Vietnam, Nepal, Northern Ireland, Ghana, Kenya, Uganda, South Africa and Israel. It has also taught TM to veterans, victims of domestic violence and abuse, soldiers and refugees suffering from PTSD, the homeless, and to American Indians, with reliably beneficial results in every area of life.

Maharishi

The history of the world shows that progress has always followed in the footsteps of those inspired individuals who have the conviction and the courage to do what they know is right. Many of these leaders, especially in the field of knowledge, had deep insights into the nature of life. They saw what everyone else saw, but in a totally new light. Copernicus observed the sun rising and setting every day, but concluded that the sun didn't move at all; it was the earth that moved around the sun. In spite of enormous resistance from scientists, religious leaders, and others, he was eventually proved correct.

Historically, it has been assumed that what cannot be conceived intellectually has no validity. This assumption has been proved false. The accepted limits of our knowledge have been superseded again and again. And as we grow in knowledge, the world takes on new dimensions; we begin to envision greater and greater possibilities. Things that were considered impossible have become not only possible but actual. In 1850, if you told a man in New York that he could step inside a container and appear in California three hours later, he would have considered you insane. Obviously, today we not only accept airplane travel as real, we accept that we can fly to the moon. What makes the "impossible" possible is knowledge. If we know the laws of gravity and jet propulsion, we can create ships that go far into space.

It was Maharishi's great genius to revive the Vedic understanding that the source of all knowledge exists in the simplest form of human awareness—pure consciousness. When we experience pure consciousness, we enliven this field of all possibilities. When we stabilize pure consciousness as a permanent reality, then literally, anything is possible.

But it is important to know that the knowledge of pure consciousness is not gained on an intellectual level. It occurs experientially, and automatically, without effort, using a simple technology. We don't have to understand all the laws of nature; we just effortlessly experience their source within our own awareness and automatically gain their support.

I have always marveled at and appreciated Maharishi's boldness in proclaiming his message of global peace and prosperity for every nation. He began as one man alone, in the late 1950s. With a simple yet powerful resolution, he traveled the globe, bringing Transcendental Meditation to millions of people across a wide spectrum of ages, educational and cultural backgrounds, with one goal—to bring peace and happiness to every single person in the world.

Notes & References

Overview

My thesis, *Physiological Effects of Transcendental Meditation: A Proposed Fourth Major State of Consciousness*, was completed in 1970 in the Department of Physiology at the University of California at Los Angeles.

An excellent review of research on neuropepodes is given by Candace Pert (1986): The Wisdom of the Receptors: Neuropepddes, The Emotions and Bodymind, *Advances*, 3(3): 8-16.

A thorough understanding of the relationship between the unified field as described in the latest theories of modern science and the field of pure consciousness as described by Maharishi's Vedic Science is given in two brilliant articles by Dr. John Hagelin (1987): Is Consciousness the Unified Field? A Field Theorist's Perspective, *Modern Science and Vedic Science*, 7(1); 29-87, and (1989) Restructuring Physics from its Foundation in Light of Maharishi's Vedic Science, *Modern Science and Vedic Science*, 3(1): 3-72.

A brief introduction to Maharishi's Vedic Science and Technology is given by Dr. Kenneth Chandler (1987) in

Modern Science and Vedic Science: An Introduction, *Modern Science and Vedic Science*, 1 (1): 5-26.

The primary works of Maharishi Mahesh Yogi in which the basic principles and technologies of the Vedic paradigm are discussed are: *Science of Being and Art of Living: Transcendental Meditation* (Plume, 2001); *On the Bhagavad-Gita: A Translation and Commentary, Chapters 1—6* (MUM Press, 2015); *Life Supported by Natural Law* (MUM Press, 1986); *Enlightenment to Every Individual and Invincibility to Every Nation* (Rheinweiler, W. Germany: Maharishi European Research University Press, 1978); *Maharishi Vedic University Inauguration* (Washington, DC: Age of Enlightenment Press, 1985); and *Maharishi's Absolute Theory of Government: Automation in Administration* (1992).

Chapter 1

A more complete understanding of the self-interacting dynamics of consciousness and the levels of the mind as explained by Maharishi is given in Life Supported by Natural Law and also in an article by Dr. Michael C. Dillbeck (1988), The Mechanics of Individual Intelligence Arising from the Field of Cosmic Intelligence—The Cosmic Psyche, *Modern Science and Vedic Science*, 2(3); 245-278.

A description of the Transcendental Meditation technique and higher states of consciousness is given in Maharishi's books: *Science of Being and Art of Living: Transcendental*

Meditation, and *On the Bhagavad-Gita: A Translation and Commentary, Chapters 1-6.*

Maurice Herzog's description of Annapurna appears in Herzofin, M. Murphy, M., White, R. A., *The Psychic Side of Sports* (Redding, MA Addison- Wesley, 1978, p. 30).

Chapter 2

Most of the original published research on the Transcendental Meditation and TM-Sidhi program is reprinted in *Scientific Research on Maharishi's Transcendental Meditation and TM-Sidhi Programme: Collected Papers,* Volumes 1-7. These are available at Maharishi University of Management Press. My original research includes several publications: Wallace, R. K. (1970), "Physiological Effects of Transcendental Meditation," *Science,* 167:1751-1754; Wallace, R. K., Benson, H., Wilson, A. F. (1971), "A Wakeful Hypometabolic Physiologic State," *American Journal of Physiology,* 221(3): 795-799; and Wallace, R. K., Benson, H. (1972), "The Physiology of Meditation," *Scientific American,* 226(2): 84-90.

A complete analysis of the research is given in The Neurophysiology of Enlightenment, MUM Press (2016). See Dr. Orme-Johnson's website TruthAboutTM.org for the most up-to-date review of research.

The passage from "Tintem Abbey" is quoted from Hayden, J. 0. (Ed.), William Wordsworth: The Poems (Vol. I), (New Haven: Yale University Press, 1981, pp 358-359).

Chapter 3

An excellent account of the story of Guillemin's and Schally's research that led to the Nobel prize is given in a three-part series in *Science* magazine (1978) by Wade, N.: Guillemin and Schally: The Years in the Wilderness, *Science*, 200: 279-282; Guillemin and Schally: The Three-Lap Race to Stockholm (ibid., pp. 411-415); and Guillemin and Schally: A Race Spurred by Rivalry (ibid., pp. 510-513).

A complete analysis of the research is given in The Neurophysiology of Enlightenment. See Dr Orme-Johnson's website truthaboutTM.org for the most up-to-date review of research.

Chapter 4

Studies on iatrogenic diseases include:

• Steel, K., Gertman, P. M., Crescenzi, C., Anderson,J. (March 12, 1981), Iatrogenic Illness on a General Medical Service at a University Hospital, *New England Journal of Medicine*, 304(11): 638-654; and

• Kramer, M. S., Hutchinson, T. A., Flegel, K. M., Naimark, L., Contardi, R., Leduc, D. G. (February 1985), Adverse Drug Reactions in General Pediatric Outpatients, *Journal of Pediatrics*, 106(2): 305-310.

The editorial, Need We Poison the Elderly So Often? is from *The Lancet*, 2(8601): 20-22, July 2, 1988.

Articles and books on problems in the treatment of heart disease include:

• Winslow, C. M., Kosecoff, J. B., Chassin, M., Kanouse, D. E., Brook, R. H. (Rand Corporation) July 22/29, 1988), The Appropriateness of Performing Coronary Artery Bypass Surgery, *Journal of the American Medical Association*, 260(4): 505-509; and

• Omish, D. et al. (1990), Can Lifestyle Changes Reverse Coronary Heart Disease? *The Lancet*, 336: 129-133.

A complete analysis of the research is given in The Neurophysiology of Enlightenment. See Dr Orme-Johnson's website truthaboutTM.org for the most up-to-date review of research.

Chapter 5

Longevity factors are discussed in Palmore, E. (Ed.), *Normal Aging II, Reports from the Duke Longitudinal Study*, 1970-1973 (Durham, NC: Duke University Press, 1974).

Research on the Transcendental Meditation and TM-Sidhi program and aging is given in *The Neurophysiology of Enlightenment* (Dharma Publications, 2015). See Dr Orme-Johnson's website truthabouttm.org for the most up-to-date review of research.

An excellent summary of Maharishi's views on aging, from which the passages from him are quoted, is given in Science, *Consciousness and Ageing: Proceedings of the Inter-*

national Conference (January 19-20, 1980), Rheinweiler, W. Germany: Maharishi European University Press.

Chapter 6

A complete analysis of the research is given in *The Neurophysiology of Enlightenment* and Dr Orme-Johnson's website truthabouttm.org for the most up-to-date review of research.

Chapter 7

Research is given in *The Neurophysiology of Enlightenment* (Dharma Publications, 2015) and Dr Orme-Johnson's website truthabouttm.org for the most up-to-date review of research.

Maharishi discusses the TM-Sidhi program and the Maharishi Effect in several publications, including *Life Supported by Natural Law, Enlightenment and Invincibility, and Maharishi's Programme to Create World Peace: Global Inauguration*, from which the passages from Maharishi are quoted.

Chapter 8

Maharishi University of Management is accredited through the PhD level. See website at mum.org for details of all programs.

Related Websites and Books

TM.org
MUM.edu
DavidLynchFoundation.org
DharmaPublications.com

An Introduction to Transcendental Meditation: Improve Your Brain Functioning, Create Ideal Health, and Gain Enlightenment Naturally, Easily, Effortlessly by Robert Keith Wallace, PhD, and Lincoln Akin Norton, Dharma Publications, 2016

The Neurophysiology of Enlightenment: How the Transcendental Meditation and TM-Sidhi Program Transform the Functioning of the Human Body, Updated and Revised by Robert Keith Wallace, PhD, Dharma Publications, 2016

Transcendence: Healing and Transformation through Transcendental Meditation by Norman Rosenthal, Tarcher/Penguin, 2011

Transcendental Meditation: Revised and Updated by Robert Roth, Primus, 1994

Science of Being and Art of Living: Transcendental Meditation by Maharishi Mahesh Yogi, Plume, 2001

Catching the Big Fish: Meditation, Consciousness, and Creativity by David Lynch, Tarcher/Penguin 2007

Dharma Parenting: Understand Your Child's Brilliant Brain for Greater Happiness, Health, Success, and Fulfillment by Robert Keith Wallace PhD, and Fredrick Travis PhD, Tarcher/Penguin, 2016

Maharishi Ayurveda and Vedic Technology: Creating Ideal Health for the Individual and World, Revised and Updated from The Physiology of Consciousness: Part 2 by Robert Keith Wallace, PhD, Dharma Publications, 2016

Dharma Health and Beauty: A User-Friendly Introduction to Ayurveda, Book One of the Smith Family Saga by Samantha Wallace with Robert Keith Wallace, PhD, Dharma Publications, 2016

The Transcendental Meditation Technique and The Journey of Enlightenment by Ann Purcell, Dragon Publishing Group, 2015

Maharishi Mahesh Yogi and His Gift to the World by William F. Sands PhD, MUM Press, 2013

Acknowledgements

I would like to acknowledge both Susan Shatkin and my wife, Samantha, for their enormous help in editing. I would also like to thank Allen Cobb for his help in preparing this book, Fran Clark for proofreading, and George Foster for his excellent cover design.

About the Author

ROBERT KEITH WALLACE is a pioneering researcher on the physiology of consciousness. His work has inspired hundreds of studies on the benefits of meditation and other mind-body techniques. Dr. Wallace's findings have been published in Science, American Journal of Physiology, and Scientific American. He received his BS in physics and his PhD in physiology from UCLA, and he conducted postgraduate research at Harvard University. Dr. Wallace is founding president and member of the board of trustees of Maharishi University of Management (MUM) in Fairfield, Iowa, He is Co-Dean of the College of Perfect Health and Professor and Chairman of the Department of Physiology and Health.

Index

A

aging 45, 51, 53, 54, 56, 57, 58, 59, 60
alcohol consumption 57
anxiety 57, 78
automatic self-transcending meditation 32

B

blood pressure 45, 57
brain imaging 32
brain wave coherence 31, 32
Brown, Calra 88

C

cardiovascular disease 57
cholesterol 57
collective consciousness 66, 67, 71, 72, 75, 80, 82, 87, 88
consciousness 1, 2, 3, 6, 8, 9, 10, 11, 14, 15, 16, 17, 18, 19, 20, 23, 24, 25, 26,
        27, 28, 29, 30, 36, 37, 38, 39, 40, 41, 45, 47, 48, 49, 51, 58, 59, 60, 63, 66,
        67, 69, 70, 71, 72, 75, 77, 80, 82, 84, 85, 87, 88, 89, 90, 101
cortisol 28
cosmic consciousness 17, 18, 19, 48

D

DNA 52, 53, 54, 59
Domash, Lawrence 63

E

EEG 74
enlightenment 14, 20, 33, 38, 59, 99
epigenetic 40

T

TM. *See* Transcendental Meditation
TM-Sidhi program 72, 73, 77
transcendental consciousness 9, 15, 17, 23, 24, 25, 26, 27, 28, 29, 30, 38, 48,
    51
Transcendental Meditation TM 2, 8, 9, 10, 16, 17, 20, 23, 26, 27, 28, 29, 32,
    33, 36, 39, 40, 47, 48, 49, 57, 58, 60, 67, 68, 69, 70, 72, 74, 76, 77, 85, 86,
    93, 95, 96, 97, 98, 100, 102, 103, 104, 105, 107, 109, 110
transcending 18, 19, 24, 30, 31, 32, 39, 47, 48

U

unified field 7, 9, 10, 11, 15, 16, 20, 58, 59, 60, 73
unity consciousness 20

V

Veda 93, 94
Vedic Science 94
Vedic tradition 2, 7, 14, 16, 60, 71, 72

W

world peace 16, 63, 69, 70, 73, 76, 82, 85, 86, 90

CPSIA information can be obtained
at www.ICGtesting.com
Printed in the USA
LVOW03s0410040817
543788LV00021B/880/P